# RISKS AND OPPORTUNITIES

## SYNTHESIS OF STUDIES ON ADOLESCENCE

Forum on Adolescence

Michele D. Kipke, *Editor*

Board on Children, Youth, and Families
Commission on Behavioral and Social Sciences and Education

National Research Council

and

Institute of Medicine

NATIONAL ACADEMY PRESS
Washington, D.C.

**NATIONAL ACADEMY PRESS**  2101 Constitution Avenue, N.W.  Washington, D.C. 20418

NOTICE:  The project that is the subject of this report was approved by the Governing Board of the National Research Council, whose members are drawn from the councils of the National Academy of Sciences, the National Academy of Engineering, and the Institute of Medicine.  The members of the committee responsible for the report were chosen for their special competences and with regard for appropriate balance.

The study was supported by Contract/Grant No. B6509 between the National Academy of Sciences and Carnegie Corporation of New York.  Any opinions, findings, conclusions, or recommendations expressed in this publication are those of the author(s) and do not necessarily reflect the view of the organizations or agencies that provided support for this project.

International Standard Book Number 0-309-06791-X

Additional copies of this report are available from National Academy Press, 2101 Constitution Avenue, N.W., Lockbox 285, Washington, D.C. 20055
Call (800) 624-6242 or (202) 334-3313 (in the Washington metropolitan area)

This report is also available on line at http://www.nap.edu

Printed in the United States of America

Suggested citation: National Research Council and Institute of Medicine (1999). "Risks and Opportunities: Synthesis of Studies on Adolescence." Forum on Adolescence. Michele D. Kipke, Editor. Board on Children, Youth, and Families. Washington, DC: National Academy Press.

# THE NATIONAL ACADEMIES

National Academy of Sciences
National Academy of Engineering
Institute of Medicine
National Research Council

The **National Academy of Sciences** is a private, nonprofit, self-perpetuating society of distinguished scholars engaged in scientific and engineering research, dedicated to the furtherance of science and technology and to their use for the general welfare. Upon the authority of the charter granted to it by the Congress in 1863, the Academy has a mandate that requires it to advise the federal government on scientific and technical matters. Dr. Bruce M. Alberts is president of the National Academy of Sciences.

The **National Academy of Engineering** was established in 1964, under the charter of the National Academy of Sciences, as a parallel organization of outstanding engineers. It is autonomous in its administration and in the selection of its members, sharing with the National Academy of Sciences the responsibility for advising the federal government. The National Academy of Engineering also sponsors engineering programs aimed at meeting national needs, encourages education and research, and recognizes the superior achievements of engineers. Dr. William A. Wulf is president of the National Academy of Engineering.

The **Institute of Medicine** was established in 1970 by the National Academy of Sciences to secure the services of eminent members of appropriate professions in the examination of policy matters pertaining to the health of the public. The Institute acts under the responsibility given to the National Academy of Sciences by its congressional charter to be an adviser to the federal government and, upon its own initiative, to identify issues of medical care, research, and education. Dr. Kenneth I. Shine is president of the Institute of Medicine.

The **National Research Council** was organized by the National Academy of Sciences in 1916 to associate the broad community of science and technology with the Academy's purposes of furthering knowledge and advising the federal government. Functioning in accordance with general policies determined by the Academy, the Council has become the principal operating agency of both the National Academy of Sciences and the National Academy of Engineering in providing services to the government, the public, and the scientific and engineering communities. The Council is administered jointly by both Academies and the Institute of Medicine. Dr. Bruce M. Alberts and Dr. William A. Wulf are chairman and vice chairman, respectively, of the National Research Council.

*v*

# Contents

# RISKS AND OPPORTUNITIES

# 1

# Introduction

Adolescents face a daunting array of developmental challenges. Beginning as early as age 9, young people experience significant physical changes as they go through puberty. Adolescents also experience emotional changes as they seek greater independence from their parents, search for acceptance by peers, and begin to navigate new adult-like roles in society. For most teenagers, these changes are accompanied by the negotiation of new and conflicting demands and pressures, the exploration of novel ideas and risky behaviors, engagement in more complex intellectual tasks, and the formation of distinct identities. At the same time, adolescence is also a time of tremendous opportunity, when parents and their teenage children can forge new, meaningful relationships and when young people can begin to serve as a resource in their communities. Throughout their development, adolescents are shaped by experiences with other individuals and in a variety of contexts and settings, including families, schools, peers, neighborhoods, community-based organizations, health care organizations, the child welfare and juvenile justice systems, the media, and others.

Our challenge as a society is to ensure that all adolescents have a promising future; find a valued place in a constructive group; learn how to form close, durable human relationships; earn a sense of worth as a person; achieve a reliable basis for making informed choices; express constructive curiosity and exploratory behavior; find ways of being useful to others; believe in a promising future with real opportunities; cultivate the inquiring and problem-solving habits of mind necessary for lifelong learning and adaptability; learn to respect democratic values and the elements of responsible citizenship; and build a healthy lifestyle. These requirements can be met only by a conjunction of the people, settings, and institutions that collectively and powerfully shape adolescent development, for better or worse.

## WEALTH OF RESEARCH

Over the past two decades, researchers have made substantial progress in describing the complexity of adolescence and in determining the common features of adolescent development. As a result, we now know how diverse and heterogeneous this age group is and how important hormonal, social, and environmental factors are in shaping their development. We also know how meaningful peers are to the formation of adolescent identity. Through this rich body of research, we have come to understand that adolescence need not be a time of turmoil and strife between teenagers and their parents, though it often is. Moreover, we now know that peer influence is not necessarily negative; rather, it can often be very positive. Finally, we now realize the significance of the settings in which adolescents grow up and how important they are to ensuring their successful transition from childhood to adulthood. The institutions within these settings—schools, health care organizations, community-based programs, and the child welfare and juvenile justice systems—need to be scrutinized carefully, as do policies designed to ensure that all adolescents grow to become healthy, happy, and productive adults.

## SCOPE OF REPORT

This report constitutes one of the first activities of the Forum on Adolescence, a cross-cutting activity of the Institute of Medicine and the National Research Council of the National Academies. Established under the auspices of the Board on Children, Youth, and Families, the forum's overarching mission is to synthesize, analyze, and evaluate scientific research on critical national issues that relate to youth and their families, as well as to disseminate research and its policy and programmatic implications. The goals of the forum are to: (1) review and establish the science base on adolescent health and development and make efforts to foster this development; (2) identify new directions and support for research in this area, approaching research as a resource to be developed cumulatively over time;

(3) showcase new research, programs, and policies that have demonstrated promise in improving the health and well-being of adolescents; (4) convene and foster collaborations among individuals who represent diverse viewpoints and backgrounds, with a view to enhancing the quality of leadership in this area; and (5) disseminate research on adolescence and its policy implications to a wide array of audiences, from the scientific community to the lay public.

The forum's mission suggested that an excellent starting point was the work already done on these topics by the National Research Council and the Institute of Medicine: nearly 60 reports published by the National Academy Press touch on adolescent issues and on issues relevant to their health and development. Taking advantage of this body of individual research syntheses, this report attempts to characterize the institution's work to date that bears on adolescence. To ensure that the data presented are reasonably up to date, this volume emphasizes reports published after 1990. Also, the reports covered address only adolescents in the United States, although the forum believes efforts are needed to understand the essential characteristics and needs of adolescents worldwide, as well as to understand which characteristics are culture specific. Each chapter concludes with a list of the reports reviewed in it. A complete list of all reports considered appears in the Appendix.

This synthesis draws from a wide range of types of reports produced by the National Academies, including committee reports that include conclusions and recommendations developed over several years, workshop reports that summarize meetings on specific topics, and other documents that reflect work carried out by experts on the topic of adolescence. Our goal in developing this synthesis on adolescence was not to produce a comprehensive or representative review of all recent research on adolescence, nor to offer conclusions or recommendations, but rather to provide a starting point for the forum's work on this important period in human development.

A number of themes emerged from our overview of the National Academies' work:

- Adolescence is a time of both tremendous opportunity and risk.
- The social context in which adolescents are developing has changed markedly during the past decade.
- Families in U.S. society have also experienced dramatic changes.
- Adolescent development does benefit from the support of a variety of social institutions.

- Specific strategies can be employed to promote the health and well-being of adolescents.
- Adolescents are increasingly joining the U.S. workforce.
- Dramatic sociodemographic changes are anticipated in the 21st century, including a great increase in the number of adolescents, as well as increasing cultural diversity within this age group.

In the pages that follow, we amplify these themes with findings gleaned from the reports examined. In only a few areas are data from outside sources incorporated into this report. These include data reported by the Bureau of the Census regarding the demographic profile of adolescents living in the United States and data reported by the U.S. Department of Health and Human Services regarding recent trends in adolescents' health and well-being. These data are included to provide a portrait of the U.S. adolescent population at the current time.

It is important to note that this report is limited in several ways. First, it does not provide, nor was it the intention to provide, a review of the science base of adolescent health and development—or to establish such a base. It provides an extensive review of certain issues, such as infection with sexually transmitted diseases and use of tobacco, alcohol, and illicit drugs, but not of others, such as motor vehicle accidents associated with alcohol use, unintended injuries, violence, and suicide.

Second, while the previously published reports focus on many of the problems and risks associated with adolescence, they do not focus equal attention on the opportunities that exist during adolescence, nor on the successes experienced by the majority of adolescents on a day-to-day basis. This exaggerated focus on the problems experienced by adolescents is due largely to the nature and types of the requests that have been directed to the National Academies by Congress, federal agencies, and private foundations. Thus, this report provides an extensive review of what can go wrong during the adolescent years and what is known about youth who are at high risk for experiencing problems and poor developmental outcomes; it does not provide this same attention to issues of resilience and what is known about adolescents who are succeeding in school, at work, and at play. Moreover, while existing reports have examined the range of factors associated with increased risks, few of them have focused on the types of interventions that have been found to be most effective at preventing or intervening when problems do occur. This report therefore runs the risk of stereotyping youth as problem-prone and problem-ridden, and potentially serves to reinforce the image that youth are a scary, troubled lot. As discussed in the concluding section, this problem-focused approach is endemic to American society, driven largely by existing program funds, which are categorical in nature and may be influenced by policies that are often inconsistent and contradictory.

Third, the connections among adolescent behaviors and the context in which they occur is missing. Thus, although adolescent problem behaviors tend to cluster, this report is structured in such a way as to treat the various problems as if they were separate from one another. While this report provides an extensive review of the various social contexts and settings that potentially influence adolescent development—such as family, community, schools, the media—there is little attention to the links between these contexts. There is also little attention to the psychological worlds of adolescents and the ways that teenagers construct and interpret the developmental changes they are experiencing, and, therefore, how the influence of social settings is mediated by psychological and cognitive processes.

In writing this report, the forum has learned a good deal about what questions have been asked about adolescents and what research has contributed to the answers. The forum has also learned what questions have not been asked and so where new efforts may be most needed. Furthermore, very recent data show evidence of an exciting and promising reversal of some trends. For example, studies suggest that an increasing number of adolescents are using condoms during sexual intercourse, and federal statistics suggest decreasing rates of unintended pregnancies among teenagers. We discuss some of these recent trends in the concluding section.

# 2

# Adolescence: A Time
of Opportunity and Risk

The demographic profile of the adolescent population has changed dramatically during the past few decades, and these changes are expected to continue well into the 21st century. Following a steady decline since the mid-1970s, the number of adolescents in the United States began to increase in the 1990s. In 1993, there were close to 36 million (35,807,000) adolescents, ages 10 to 19, representing nearly 14 percent of the population. This increase is expected to continue until the year 2020, gradually leveling off between the years 2020 and 2050 (Figure 2-1). Until recently, more of the adolescent population consisted of younger people: 52 percent (18,529,000) between ages 10 and 14, compared with 48 percent (17,278,000) between ages 15 and 19. As of 1990, however, this pattern was reversed: 49 percent of adolescents between ages 10 and 14 and 51 percent between ages 15 and 19. This trend is also likely to continue into the 21st century, and increasingly researchers, service providers, and policy makers are arguing that the age frame that defines adolescence should include youth up to age 24. In terms of this new definition, a very different profile emerges with respect to future population projections: the adolescent and young adult population will continue to increase well beyond the year 2050 (Figure 2-1).

In addition, the increasing racial and ethnic diversity in the general population of the United States has resulted in increasing proportions of adolescents belonging to racial and ethnic minority groups. Although 74 percent of all children in the United States in 1980 were white, this propor-

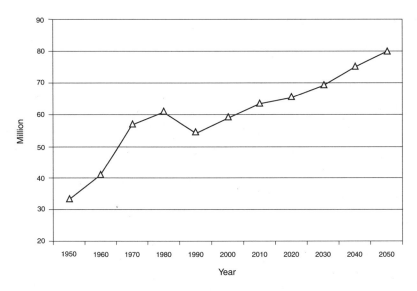

FIGURE 2-1 Number of youth ages 10-24 selected years, 1950-1990, and projected, 2000-2050. SOURCE: Data from Bureau of the Census (1965, 1974, 1982, 1996, 1999).

tion has steadily decreased ever since and is projected to continue to have a downward trend through the year 2050 (Figure 2-2). In 1993, more than one-third of the population of adolescents ages 10 to 19 were Hispanic or nonwhite. Black children were the largest minority population prior to 1997, but now their numbers are slightly superseded by Hispanic children (each making up about 15 percent of the total child population). The U.S. Bureau of Census is estimating that by the year 2020, more than one in five U.S. children will be Hispanic. The Asian population will also continue its rapid increase, from 4 to 6 percent by the year 2020. This rapid rise in racial and ethnic diversity in the United States is expected to continue through the coming decades.

## THE DEVELOPING ADOLESCENT

Adolescence is one of the most fascinating and complex transitions in the life span: a time of accelerated growth and change, second only to infancy; a time of expanding horizons, self-discovery, and emerging independence; a time of metamorphosis from childhood to adulthood. Its begin-

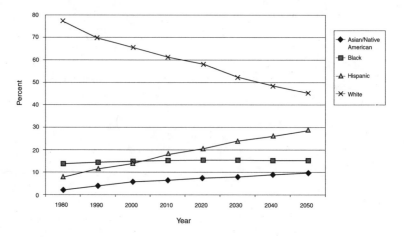

**FIGURE 2-2** Percentage distribution of children ages 10-24 in the United States selected years, 1980-1990, and projected 2000-2050. SOURCE: Data from Bureau of the Census (1965, 1974, 1982, 1996, 1999).

ning is associated with biological, physical, behavioral, and social transformations that roughly correspond to the move from elementary school to middle or junior high school. The events of this crucial formative phase can shape an individual's life course—and, by extension, an entire society.

In the United States, the period called adolescence is considered to extend over many years, so it can be usefully subdivided into three developmental phases. Early adolescence encompasses the biological changes of puberty as well as sexual and psychological awakenings, extending roughly from ages 10 through 14. Middle adolescence is a time of increased autonomy and experimentation, covering ages 15 to 17. Late adolescence, for those who delay their entry into adult roles because of educational or social factors, can stretch from age 18 into the early 20s. Each phase has a unique set of developmental challenges, opportunities, and risks.

Puberty is often used to define the onset of early adolescence. Triggered by preprogrammed events in the brain, the pituitary gland produces hormones that in turn stimulate the secretion of sex hormones. These hormones have powerful effects on many tissues of the body, including the brain, and lead to significant changes in social, emotional, and sexual behavior. Although the biology of puberty has remained essentially the same for many generations, the social context in which these biological events occur has changed dramatically. Institutionalization, urbanization, technological advances, geographic mobility, and cultural diversity have radically transformed the world, and the interaction between biology and this new environment has fundamentally altered the circumstances of growing up as an adolescent in the United States.

Over the past two decades, the research base in the field of adolescent development has undergone a growth spurt, and knowledge has expanded significantly. New studies have allowed more complex views of the multiple dimensions of adolescence, fresh insights into the process and timing of puberty, and new perspectives on the behaviors associated with the second decade of life. At the same time, the field's underlying theoretical assumptions have changed and matured.

For much of this century, scientists and scholars tended to assume that the changes associated with adolescence were almost entirely dictated by biological influences. It has been viewed as a time of storm and stress, best contained or passed through as quickly as possible. *Adolescence*, a 1904 book by G. Stanley Hall, typified this standpoint. It was Hall who popularized the notion that adolescence is inevitably a time of psychological and emotional turmoil. Half a century later, psychoanalytic writers including Anna Freud accepted and augmented Hall's emphasis on turmoil. Even today, "raging hormones" continue to be a popular explanation for the lability, aggression, and sexual activity associated with adolescence. Intense conflict between adolescents and their parents is often considered an unavoidable consequence of adolescence. However, this assumption has not been supported by scientific evidence. The assumption that turmoil and conflict are inevitable consequences of the teenage years may even have prevented some adolescents from receiving the support and services they needed.

Research is now creating a more realistic view of adolescence. Adolescence continues to be seen as a period of time encompassing difficult developmental challenges, but there is wider recognition that biology is only one factor that affects young people's development, adjustment, and behavior. There is mounting evidence to suggest that the adolescent years need not be troubled ones. There is now greater recognition that most young people move through the adolescent years without experiencing great trauma or getting into serious trouble. Although adolescence can certainly be a challenging span of years, individuals negotiate it with varying degrees of difficulty, just as they do other periods of life. Moreover, when problems do arise during adolescence, they should not be considered "normal"—i.e., that the adolescent will grow out of them—nor should they be ignored. Indeed, parents, teachers, members of the community, service providers, and social institutions can both promote healthy development among adolescents and intervene effectively when problems do arise.

There is also a growing recognition that only a segment of the adolescent population is at high risk for experiencing serious problems. Over the past 50 years, studies conducted in North America and Europe have documented that only about a quarter of the adolescent population is at high risk for, or especially vulnerable to, experiencing psychosocial problems and poor developmental outcomes, such as academic failure and school drop-out, alcohol and other drug abuse, delinquency and problems with the law, and violence. These adolescents are not believed to be at increased risk because of biological or hormonal changes associated with puberty, but rather from a complex interaction among biological, environmental, and social factors. Indeed, there is mounting evidence that most biological changes interact with a wide range of contextual, psychological, social, and environmental factors that affect behavior.

Adolescence is frequently described as a time of increased risk-taking. This is in part due to the fact that adolescence is developmentally a time when teenagers begin to experiment with tobacco, alcohol, and other drugs and initiate sexual intercourse (as many as two-thirds reporting initiating sexual intercourse before graduating from high school). It is also because the outcomes associated with some of these behaviors can be so disastrous: the rates of many sexually transmitted diseases are highest during the adolescent and young adult years; many adolescents experience unintended pregnancies, which can significantly affect their life course and limit future opportunities; a disproportionately high number of automobile accidents occurs among teenagers, and typically alcohol is involved; and violence has increased to the point that homicide is the second leading cause of death among young people.

As children develop into adolescents, they gain greater autonomy and are exposed to a greater variety of adults and peers. They therefore begin to have more opportunities to make choices about who they will spend time with and how they will behave.

Adolescents' involvement in risk-taking behaviors has been explained in a number of ways. Some teenagers tend to be especially high in sensation-seeking, while others use these behaviors to appear more mature or because of heightened egocentrism. Increasingly, researchers attribute these behaviors to a combination of individual, social, and environmental factors. One of the factors that has received much less attention in recent years is adolescent decision making. In fact, most research conducted on decision-making processes has been carried out with adults.

Decision making involves not only recognizing consequences, but also determining the likelihood that a consequence will occur. Adolescents' involvement in risky behaviors has often been attributed to their thinking of themselves as invulnerable—as thinking that bad consequences will not happen to them. Research now shows that adolescents are no more likely than adults to see themselves as invulnerable. That is not to say that adults do a good job of estimating probabilities of the likelihood of their experiencing negative consequences. Numerous studies have found that adults tend to see themselves as less likely than others to experience negative outcomes and more likely to experience positive ones. Young people favor their own experience and anecdotal evidence over probabilistic information in making decisions, particularly about social situations, as do adults. Adolescents also make important decisions under a set of circumstances in which we know adults have difficulty: unfamiliar tasks, choices with uncertain outcomes, and ambiguous situations.

Adolescents' social cognition—the way they think about their social world, the people they interact with, and the groups they participate in— differs from that of adults and influences their decision-making skills.

Emotions affect how people think and behave and influence the information they attend to. When people are experiencing positive emotions, they tend to underestimate the likelihood of negative consequences to their actions; when they are experiencing negative emotions, they tend to focus on the near term and lose sight of the big picture. Both adolescents' and adults' decision-making abilities are influenced by emotions. However, there is evidence that adolescents experience more intense emotions than adults, which suggests that they may process information differently and therefore make different decisions than adults do.

## SOCIAL CONTEXT
## IN WHICH ADOLESCENTS DEVELOP

One of the important insights to emerge from scientific inquiry into adolescence in the past two decades is that problem behaviors, as well as health-enhancing ones, tend to cluster in the same individual, and these behaviors tend to reinforce one another. Crime, dropping out of school, teenage pregnancy and childbearing, and drug abuse typically are considered separately, but in the real world they often occur together. Teenagers who drink and smoke are more likely to initiate sex earlier than their peers; those who engage in these behavior patterns often have a history of difficulties in school. The fact that the health-enhancing behaviors cluster together suggests that families, schools, and other social institutions have an important opportunity to foster healthy lifestyles during adolescence by addressing common roots of both positive and negative behaviors.

Another important insight of scientific inquiry is the profound influence of settings on adolescents' behavior and development. Until recently, research conducted to understand adolescent behavior, particularly risk-related behaviors, focused on the individual characteristics of teenagers and their families. A 1993 National Research Council study took a critical look at how families, communities, and other institutions are serving the needs of youth in the United States. This study concluded that adolescents depend not only on their families, but also on the neighborhoods in which they live, the schools that they attend, the health care system, and the workplace from which they learn a wide range of important skills. If sufficiently enriched, all of these settings and social institutions in concert can help teenagers successfully make the transition from childhood to adulthood.

Yet the unfortunate reality is that in the United States, these settings and social institutions are under severe stress. It is now not unusual for families to be headed either by a single mother or by two wage earners, and as much as 40 percent of young adolescents' time is unstructured, unsupervised, and consequently unproductive; much of this time occurs during the after-school hours when adolescents are frequently alone, watching television. Neighborhoods and communities—particularly inner-city, poor neighborhoods—are also increasingly less able to provide resources and services to youth, and school systems are often not organized to provide opportunities to learn and grow during the after-school hours.

In the past few decades, researchers have started to examine why some adolescents in low-income communities successfully navigate environmental challenges, while others, similarly situated, adopt lifestyles characterized by drug use, unprotected sexual behavior, dropping out of school, delinquency, gang membership, and violence. Researchers have also sought to identify not only risk factors that may be associated with these problems, but also patterns of resilience that protect teens and encourage them to succeed. This research has emphasized the need to examine the "whole" youth—a concept that describes the assets as well as the deficits of individual adolescents—rather than isolating selected problem behaviors associated with adolescents in difficult circumstances. This research has also attempted to take a broader view of development by not focusing on each critical developmental stage in isolation from one another but rather to look at development across the life span—from early childhood to the middle childhood years, adolescence, and adulthood. This is largely because of the growing literature that suggests that problems experienced later in life are typically foreshadowed by problems that occurred earlier in life.

Although this focus on the whole youth has been applauded, much more work needs to be done before the picture is clear about which combination of factors, influences, contexts, and interventions will ultimately ensure the healthy development of children and adolescents.

## CHANGES IN U.S. FAMILIES

Years of research have shown that adolescents are most likely to develop into healthy, happy, and productive adults when they are supported by a caring family. Such a positive environment is characterized by nurturing and mutual respect and by the serious and sustained interest of parents in the lives of their adolescent children.

Contrary to popular belief, adolescence is a time when many young people continue to need more parental attention. They need guidance and close supervision. They need a parent or other responsible adult to listen and respond to them as they shape their ideas. They need help with setting goals. And they still need to be taught ethical behavior and the appropriate ways of handling conflict with others. Parents who offer this type of support to their adolescent children can provide powerful protection against the possibility that they may engage in unhealthy practices, become socially isolated, or become troubled or depressed.

Today, adolescents are growing up in families that are diverse with respect to their size, shape, and structure. From families characterized as traditional with two parents and a stay-at-home mother, which was typical in the 1950s and 1960s, to the dual-career families and stepfamilies that gained in prominence in the late 1980s and 1990s, today there is no typical or normative family setting in which adolescents grow and develop.

In addition, changing societal and economic factors have threatened the stability of many families in today's society. Many of these changes have occurred during the past 30 years, including increased rates of divorce, increases in the number of single parents, increases in the rate of mothers' employment, and increases in the proportion of families living in poverty. For example, by the early 1990s, nearly half of all marriages ended in divorce, a rate twice that of 1960, and about a quarter of all births were to unmarried women. The net result has been that nearly 25 percent of all children live with only one parent, usually the mother, a rate double that of 1970. Overall, about 50 percent of all children today will reside in a single-parent home before age 18, spending an average of 6 years with a single parent. These changes have transformed the nature of family life, as well as the experiences of adolescents.

Although there has been less research than the issue deserves, many argue that the time that American children spend with their parents has decreased significantly during the past few decades. Under the best of circumstances, raising a child is a difficult experience, but during this past decade, as more families are defined as dual-income and single-parent households, parent spend on average 11 fewer hours with their children each week compared with parents in 1960. In addition, less than 5 percent of all families have another adult (such as a grandparent) living in the home, compared with 50 percent two generations ago. This reduces the backup support that might otherwise be available to working parents. It is also a commonly held belief that as parents spend less time with their children, they have less time available to provide guidance and supervision, and fewer opportunities to instill values. More research is needed, however, to determine if in fact it is true that parents are spending less time with their teens, and what impact this has on the safety, security, and well-being of today's adolescents.

One of the most profound changes in the past few decades is the increased proportion of adolescents living in or near poverty. Patterns in family structure are associated with differential economic status, with households headed by two parents reporting significantly higher incomes than those headed by single parents. In 1993, the median household income for adolescents (ages 12 to 17) living with one parent was $38,935, 18 percent lower than that for adolescents living with both parents. Twice as many one-parent families lived below the poverty line (16.8 percent compared with 8.4 percent for two-parent families). This disparity is more dramatic for one-parent households headed by women: the median family income for adolescents in these settings was $15,837, and 42 percent lived below the poverty line. Female-headed households experience greater poverty due to a variety of factors, including pay inequities faced by women and lack of paternal financial support.

Among the many factors that influence adolescents' health, development, and well-being, perhaps the most powerful is family income. Decisions about housing, neighborhoods, schools, and social opportunities for adolescents are largely controlled by income. A family's income and employment status also strongly influence its access to health care services and the quality of those services. Opportunities for advanced education and training and entry into the workforce are also closely linked to family income. On a more fundamental level, income is a powerful influence in shaping the most important of settings, the family itself. There is evidence that economic hardship—whether from low wages, sustained poverty, or unemployment—significantly diminishes the emotional well-being of parents, with direct and indirect effects on their children's health and well-being. Thus, the decline in economic security of young families has had important and far-reaching consequences for many children and adolescents.

Divorce has added an even more challenging dimension to the problems of today's families. Children from divorced families must confront the emotional stress of a breakup—the often prolonged time preceding and subsequent to divorce proceedings—in addition to conditions associated with single parenthood. Many of these children experience elevated levels of depression and anger and declining school performance and self-esteem. Children of divorce experience a range of stresses of greater magnitude than children in two-parent households, and these stresses are directly associated with adolescents' involvement in behaviors that may be associated with poor developmental outcomes. Adolescents who experienced divorce at an early age may be at particularly high risk of school failure and problems with emotional adjustment.

When custodial parents remarry, children often experience another stressful transition, which appears to be especially difficult for adolescent girls. This effect is diminished, however, when separated parents maintain collegial relations and engage in cooperative parenting.

While it is certainly not the case that all adolescents growing up in poor or divorced families are destined to problems and failure, there is an extensive literature that suggests that adolescents living in families experiencing economic hardship, divorce, or both are at increased risk for a range of health and behavioral problems, including school failure, use and abuse of alcohol and other drugs, unintended pregnancies, and illegal activities. The effects of these challenges can be moderated, however, by parents' behaviors. Parents who maintain strong emotional relationships with their children, display supportive attitudes, and practice loving, warm, yet firm and consistent parenting can help their children and adolescents cope more successfully.

Despite these changes in the structure and composition of families, it remains the case that the family remains an extremely important influence on adolescents, and having a positive and warm relationship with parents remains one of the most important predictors of healthy, secure development during the adolescent years.


## PEER RELATIONSHIPS

Adolescents spend twice as much time with peers than with parents or other adults, and adolescent peer groups function with much less adult supervision than do childhood peer groups. The relative importance of peer group influence versus family influence on adolescents has been the subject of controversy. The popular notion of the reluctant teenager being pressured into trying a risky behavior by friends may be overly simplistic. It appears that adolescents select their closest friends on the basis of similar interests, as do adults; young people tend to have two to four best friends who are very similar to themselves. It is unusual for a young person who does not use cigarettes or alcohol to select a close friend who does use them. Even if the adolescent has a friend who behaves differently, for example, the nonsmoking teenager who has a friend who smokes cigarettes, it appears that peer influence is relatively small and mediated by family factors, such as parental monitoring. Some research suggests that peer pressure accounts for between 10 and 40 percent of the variations in adolescents' smoking and drinking behavior. Other research has found that susceptibility to peer influence may be higher among younger teenagers than older teenagers and is negatively correlated with their confidence in their social skills.

The influence peers exert can be indirect or passive. Indeed, young people are sometimes influenced as much by what they think their peers are doing as by what they really are doing. A young person may think that everyone is smoking or everyone is sexually active and may therefore feel pressure to try those behaviors.

## REPORTS REFERENCED

- *Adolescent Behavior and Health* (1978)
- *Adolescent Decision Making: Implications for Prevention Programs* (1999)
- *Adolescent Development and the Biology of Puberty: Summary of a Workshop on New Research* (1999)
- *America's Fathers and Public Policy* (1994)
- *Inner-City Poverty in the United States* (1990)
- *Integrating Federal Statistics on Children: Report of a Workshop* (1995)
- *Losing Generations: Adolescents in High-Risk Settings* (1993)
- *Reducing Risks for Mental Disorders: Frontiers for Preventive Intervention Research* (1994)
- *Violence and the American Family* (1994)
- *Violence in Families: Assessing Prevention and Treatment Programs* (1998)
- *Youth Development and Neighborhood Influences: Challenges and Opportunities* (1996)

# 3

# Supporting Adolescents
# with Social Institutions

Communities and institutions that surround adolescents are increasingly challenged by the changing social and economic conditions in society. These conditions include the decline in economic security for poor and middle-class families, the increase in the number of single-parent households, and the rise in the number of neighborhoods with concentrated poverty that are spatially and socially isolated from middle- and working-class areas. Such trends place enormous stresses on public and private institutions—neighborhoods, schools, the health care delivery system, the workplace, and employment and training centers. For adolescents to be successful in a society that offers many choices and challenges, it is abundantly clear that they need support from all the settings and social institutions that make up a community.

## NEIGHBORHOODS AND COMMUNITY SETTINGS

Most of the social interactions of families and adolescents are embedded within neighborhood settings. A neighborhood can be defined both spatially, as a geographic area, and functionally, as a set of social networks. However defined, neighborhood is a key setting for adolescent development. Neighborhood characteristics are increasingly viewed as part of the broader range of influences that can affect adolescents, although the magnitude of their impact is uncertain and difficult to measure. Neighborhood factors that influence adolescent health, development, and well-being include:

- the decline in economic security (including decreasing real earnings and rising levels of unemployment), especially for young adults;
- the increase in single-parent, usually female-headed, families;
- the relation of male joblessness to social disorganization and rational planning for families and adolescents;
- easy access to illegal drugs and guns;
- high rates of youth crime and juvenile detention; and
- the role of illegal or underground economies in providing for basic goods and services.

These factors contribute to the absence of adult supervision and monitoring, a dearth of safe places to gather, the absence of constructive activities during idle periods, increased exposure to law enforcement and prison settings, and diminished opportunities for interaction with positive role models and needed institutional resources.

Patterns of residential transience, often generated by poverty, represent another neighborhood factor that can influence youth development. Frequent household moves, disruptions in daily routines caused by unrelated individuals entering or departing the household, and mobility among neighbors can undermine community ties, weaken support networks, and reduce privacy. However, such transience does not inevitably disrupt development if adolescents have opportunities to sustain relationships with trusted adults.

Encounters with neighborhoods are shaped not only by parenting processes and children's experiences, but also by class, gender, and ethnicity. There is a great deal of evidence that suggests that social class influences the character of the neighborhood organization and culture. For example, many poor adolescents are growing up in racially segregated and economically isolated neighborhoods. In these neighborhoods, a high proportion of adults are poor, unemployed, on welfare, or single parents. Research shows that these adolescents are in fact at increased risk for school failure and dropping out of school, unintended pregnancy, abuse of alcohol and other drugs, delinquency, and victimization and perpetration of violence. The strength and quality of social networks in neighborhoods also may affect the types of adult interactions that adolescents experience, which in turn can influence their choice of role models and life course options.

The child's age and gender are also likely to result in sharply divergent experiences that modify the impact of neighborhoods on development. Girls typically are granted less autonomy and are subject to greater parental control. Especially in low-income areas, boys often spend more time hanging out on the streets, and at younger ages. Thus, neighborhood influences may operate differently for different age groups by gender.

A missing factor in the lives of adolescents in disadvantaged communities, especially black adolescents, is exposure to successful, upwardly mobile adults. Far too often, adults who become successful move out of the disadvantaged areas to higher-income urban or suburban communities. Lacking this exposure, adolescents in disadvantaged neighborhoods may have limited opportunities to learn about strategies for family financial planning, balancing work and child care responsibilities, and identifying educational and career opportunities across the life span.

Research on social settings has increasingly called attention to the role of the unrelated adults who come into contact with adolescents in neighborhood and other social settings. They include teachers, mentors, coaches, employers, religious leaders, service providers, shop owners, and community leaders who may influence youth perceptions and behavior in their everyday settings. Researchers are exploring how the absence or presence of these individuals affects adolescents' perceptions of their own potential contributions and life options.

Despite findings from the growing literature suggesting the importance of neighborhood influences on adolescent development, the evidence for direct neighborhood effects is weak and often inconsistent. Moreover, it is not clear how community resources translate into opportunities for families and their children. Research is therefore needed to better characterize the ways in which neighborhoods influence both negative and positive developmental outcomes among children and adolescents, as well as the ways in which neighborhood influences, economic influences, family influences, and other social resources collectively interact with one another to influence the development of children and adolescents. Research is also needed to help explain why some children and adolescents are more resilient than others in adverse situations, and what combination of factors serve to buffer against negative or potentially harmful influences.

## SCHOOLS

Today, virtually all teenagers in the United States are enrolled in school; this is in stark contrast to 50 years ago when fewer than half of adolescents were enrolled in school. Students now spend more time in school (i.e., number of days) and remain in school for more years than they did in previous decades. While at the turn of the century high schools were intended for the elite, today the American education system is intended to meet the needs of a diverse and growing population. In addition, it is expected to provide youth with the knowledge, skills, and credentials needed for adulthood in modern society. Education is often considered the ticket out of poverty for children growing up in disadvantaged neighborhoods. For many adolescents, however, schools do not serve these functions nor do they successfully meet these needs, despite years of public debate and numerous efforts at school reform.

Indeed, in recent years, there has been much debate about how to structure schools for young adolescents, given that students face two major school transitions during adolescence—moving from elementary school to the middle grades and, two or three years later, moving to high school. Each transition dramatically changes their educational experiences. As they move through the education system, students face increasing complexity: compared with elementary schools, middle and senior school facilities and the student body tend to be larger; they are more likely to use competitive motivational strategies; there is greater rigor in grading and an increased focus on normative grading standards; there is greater teacher control; and instruction is delivered to the entire classroom rather than to individuals or smaller clusters of students. These changes can be stressful for some adolescents, and research indicates that the experience of transition itself may have an independent negative effect on students' attitudes and achievement, especially in large urban schools. It is important to note that although some aspects of the transition into middle and high school may be difficult for students to negotiate, not all students experience the same degree of stress during these transitions.

With each transition to a new school, more stratification occurs. Different teachers teach different subjects, and, within subject matter, students are often grouped by ability level. This grouping of students according to perceived ability is called tracking. Students placed in the lower tracks are at the greatest risk for being retained in a grade, and, by the same token, students who repeat a grade are likely to be placed in the lower tracks. The practices of tracking and grade retention are both grounded in tradition; they are intended to ensure that instruction is paced at students' ability to learn and that subjects are mastered before a student advances. An unintended consequence for some students is that they feel stigmatized: separated from many of their peers, they may develop a sense of uncertainty and alienation toward school. More significantly, tracking and grade retention may imperil students' academic achievement.

Because of stratification by social class and residence, students from poor families often receive their education in the poorest schools. These schools usually have fewer financial and material resources, and they often are unable to retain the most skilled administrators and teachers. Student achievement levels in these schools are significantly lower on virtually all measures than those of students in suburban schools.

Compensatory education funds from federal and state sources are targeted toward disadvantaged and low-achieving students, but they have shown limited success, particularly among older adolescents. Dropout prevention programs for older adolescents are less effective when implemented as remedial or vocational add-ons to the regular curriculum. It has become apparent that the roots of poor achievement lie not only in the conditions of poverty or in individual differences, but also in the use of such instructional practices as tracking and grade retention, and the generally lower expectations for adolescents in schools in lower-income communities.

Despite these shortcomings of today's educational system, it is clear that adolescents who complete high school are better off than those who drop out, not only in terms of earnings but also in terms of cognitive development. While much less is known about the impact of schools on adolescents' psychosocial development, it is clear that adolescents who drop out of school are at very high risk for problems, including (but not limited to) alcohol and other drug abuse, delinquency and involvement in criminal behavior, unintended pregnancies, and prematurely leaving or running away from home.

Increasingly, schools are being transformed as community-based settings in which primary health and mental health services are being delivered, including prevention and health promotion interventions targeting a wide range of behaviors. In the past, school health officials focused on the prevention of infectious diseases, such as tuberculosis and chicken pox. Today schools seek to prevent or address a wide spectrum of health concerns, ranging from violence to substance abuse, risky sexual behaviors, tobacco use, inadequate physical activity, and poor dietary habits—the six issues at the core of 70 percent of all adolescent health problems, according to the Centers for Disease Control and Prevention. Many schools have turned to a comprehensive health program that integrates age-appropriate health education courses with physical education, course work in nutrition, health and psychological services, counseling, and other related services.

Although they may take many forms, comprehensive school health programs are characterized by complementary strategies, activities, and services designed to promote the optimal physical, emotional, social, and educational development of students.

Increasingly, schools are also developing school-based or school-linked health care services as well as partnering with other community-based social service programs to offer students comprehensive primary health care and preventive services. Since they first were conceived, however, these programs have been hampered by poor coordination, inadequate or unreliable funding, and a lack of knowledge about the effectiveness of behavioral interventions. While many of the components needed to create a comprehensive service delivery system of care are in place in many communities, the schools and these communities often lack an infrastructure to facilitate coordination; in these cases, fragmentation of resources has generally limited their growth.

## HEALTH CARE DELIVERY SYSTEM

During the past two decades, the field of adolescent health care has grown rapidly, as health care providers and health educators have come to better understand that the health care needs of teenagers are quite different from those of children and adults.

There is consensus that the most significant threats to the health of today's adolescents are behavioral in nature and associated with psychosocial risks rather than natural causes. Unlike children and adults, adolescents are less vulnerable to disease or illness (e.g., cancer, infectious diseases, genetic or congenital diseases) and more vulnerable to death from injury, homicide, and suicide than any other age group, and this risk has been increasing during the past several decades. Other health problems include alcohol and drug abuse, infection with sexually transmitted diseases, unintended pregnancy and its outcomes, mental health problems (e.g., lack of self-esteem, depression, suicide), and physical and sexual abuse.

In this area there are two important points to make. First, the leading causes of morbidity and mortality among adolescents are behavioral in nature, all are almost entirely preventable, and they have resulted in a movement away from traditional medical models that emphasize assessment, diagnosis, and treatment of diseases to a health promotion model. Health promotion involves screening for psychosocial and behavioral risk factors in an effort to prevent youth from engaging in risk behaviors. Adolescent health care providers now also encourage healthy lifestyle patterns with respect to diet, exercise, and sleep in part because these behaviors are likely to persist into adulthood. The second important point to make is that health care providers now recognize that interventions introduced during the adolescent years could very well affect health outcomes during the adult and senior years. Indeed, it is now widely believed that adolescence is an important time to intervene in an effort to encourage people to adopt a healthy lifestyle that they may very well maintain into the adult years.

Despite the recognized importance of providing these services to adolescents, many of them lack a consistent source of basic care over time. They are far less likely to visit a doctor's office or to have any regular source of medical care than are either young children or adults. Many of their health issues, such as drug use and sexual intercourse, are socially stigmatizing or difficult to discuss. Such issues make physician-patient relations particularly difficult; adolescents may be unwilling to discuss or deal with these problems in hospital-based or outpatient clinic-based health care delivery settings.

The failure of the U.S. health care system to address the needs of adolescents is especially acute for those who engage in high-risk behavior. Few physicians specialize in adolescent health, and other practitioners are poorly trained to recognize or deal with adolescent health problems, particularly when the symptoms are psychosocial rather than physical in nature. The overall system is fragmented, which is a particular problem for adolescents because of the diversity of their needs. For many adolescents, the health care system lacks all of the essential elements of primary care: a consistent point of entry into the system, a locus of ongoing responsibility, adequate backup for consultation and referral services by adolescent specialists, and comprehensiveness.

Adolescents from low-income families—precisely those who are at highest risk for health problems—are also those least likely to be covered by health insurance. Insurance coverage is the major determinant of whether children or adolescents have access to health care. This finding is consistent across many studies: compared with children who have insurance coverage, uninsured children have many unmet health care needs. As many as a quarter of adolescents are thought to have no health insurance benefits. Even when available, insurance may be inadequate for the many needs of adolescents. Most private plans emphasize treatment rather than prevention or outreach, and payment restrictions (maximums, coinsurance, deductibles) further reduce the range of services available. Moreover, the amounts and services covered by Medicaid vary widely from state to state, and in some states Medicaid does not even provide coverage for adolescents; complicated regulations may also discourage adolescents from seeking care. Rules regarding parental notification, which have a deterrent effect in the case of contraceptive use and abortion, may also deter adolescents from seeking other health care services. Inadequate reimbursement schedules may cause providers to limit the number of Medicaid patients that they will serve.

Mental health services share many of these same problems. It has been estimated that approximately 25 percent of all adolescents have a significant mental health problem, yet the mental health system is designed to serve only a few, select adolescents; these services typically are provided through special education in schools, community mental health centers, and inpatient facilities; the services are rarely integrated and are often unavailable to the adolescents who need them most. In short, the mental health system meets the needs of only a small minority of adolescents.

Mental health services have also traditionally focused on treatment rather than prevention or mental health promotion. Even for young people with insurance benefits, mental health treatment often is offered on a short-term basis, in restrictive inpatient settings. In schools, less than one-third of all students in special education receive psychological, social work, or counseling services. Only about 2 percent of all adolescents receive service from a school psychologist; there is only one school psychologist per 2,500 students nationwide. When mental health services are offered, they have been focused on preventing behavioral problems such as substance abuse, violence, and delinquency, rather than on promoting emotional well-being.

Children's health insurance became a subject of national debate early in 1997 when President Clinton and members of Congress began to develop a variety of competing proposals to expand coverage for children. After several months of active discussion and negotiation, Congress enacted the State Children's Health Insurance Program (SCHIP) as part of the Balanced Budget Act of 1997. With SCHIP, $24 billion of new funding is available to states over five years, including $20.3 billion for new initiatives based on private insurance coverage and $3.6 billion for Medicaid improvements. States may use SCHIP funds to broaden their Medicaid programs, to start up or expand state-sponsored or private insurance programs, or to support a combination of programs. The potential for flexibility in SCHIP designs appeals to most states because it gives them the opportunity to provide coverage and services in ways that reflect the state's unique circumstances and characteristics, such as the availability of insurance products and providers, the geographic distribution of uninsured children, and the potential sources of financing, among others.

This flexibility also raises some technical and practical issues. The most fundamental question is this: With so much variation possible, how will we know whether SCHIP is effective? Unless there is consistent reporting of reliable data within and across states, it will be difficult to evaluate the program's impact. At this very early stage in the program, it is vitally important to design and develop systems of accountability and to anticipate needs for information and communication based on experiences with other national and state programs, especially those that involve low-income working families.

It is too early to tell what impact SCHIP will have on the health and well-being of children and adolescents. Over the next several years, however, it will be important to measure the extent to which the new children's health insurance programs alleviate the pressure on other sources of funding for uncompensated care. Unless better data systems are developed, this will be extremely difficult to measure. Thus, the advent of the SCHIP program offers a unique opportunity to track and measure changes in the number of uninsured children and to assess the program's effectiveness from its onset. Lessons learned from the evaluation of the program will have important implications for the likelihood and nature of future insurance expansions.

## CHILD WELFARE AND JUVENILE JUSTICE

For many adolescents who enter its care, the child welfare system has become a high-risk setting. Demographic trends and the efforts aimed at deinstitutionalization in the 1970s and at community-based service alternatives in the early 1980s temporarily reduced the number of adolescents in the child welfare system, but by the mid-1980s the trend was reversed. Whether factors outside the service system, such as increased poverty and broken families, overwhelmed efforts to develop community service alternatives is not clear, but what is evident is that the system was not designed to address the challenges presented by troubled teens.

A large number of adolescents become part of the child welfare system while still living in their parents' homes. They often come into the system because they are abused or neglected or because they are a sibling of a younger child who has been abused or neglected. Services may be provided to small children and their parents, but it is unusual for adolescents to receive services. Many parents receive homemaker services and parent-training classes, for instance, and young children may receive day care services. But it is generally believed that the problems of adolescents will be resolved when a parent changes his or her behavior or when some of the stresses in a parent's life are relieved.

Many professionals have observed that there are actually two child welfare systems—one for young children and another for adolescents. Although the system for young children is viewed as deeply flawed, the system for adolescents has even more complex and formidable problems. One example is the recruiting and retaining of foster parents. It is particularly difficult to find foster parents for adolescents, for whom family life is often a source of conflict and whose behaviors may be both destructive and difficult to control. Hence, it is often necessary to place adolescents in more restrictive living arrangements like group homes and residential treatment centers.

Since the mid-1970s, the federal government and the states have sought noncorrectional alternatives for adolescents who engage in antisocial but not serious criminal activities. These adolescents were typically classified as "minors in need of supervision," but they are neither treated as offenders nor incarcerated. A number of alternatives to community-based services have arisen to serve them.[1] Delinquent adolescents who were once in the child welfare system now often shuttle between systems: detention or correctional centers operated by juvenile courts and correctional departments, on one hand, and group homes, residential treatment facilities, and halfway houses operated by the child welfare or mental health system, on the other. For adolescents who engage in more serious crimes, the corrections system then becomes the custodial parent.

Both the juvenile and the adult criminal justice systems are generally failing in their efforts to rehabilitate offenders. The decline in confidence in the effectiveness of rehabilitation and escalating rates of imprisonment

---

[1]The findings from these noncorrectional alternatives have not been discussed in published National Research Council and Institute of Medicine reports. However, a report synthesizing the findings of programs targeted to youth within the juvenile justice system, as well as other research findings regarding juvenile crime, is currently scheduled to be completed by the Panel on Juvenile Crime of the Committee on Law and Justice in 2000.

mean that adolescents caught in the juvenile and the adult criminal justice systems may live adult lives marked by unemployment, low-paying jobs, ill health, and crime.

The juvenile justice system that emerged early in this century not only included training and reform schools and other forms of institutionalization, but it also made frequent use of suspended sentences and probation. Now the juvenile justice system has many of the adversarial and punitive characteristics of the adult system. The shift from an earlier emphasis on rehabilitation and treatment to the current emphasis on punishment has had important consequences for the sentencing and punishment of young offenders.

Black and Hispanic adolescents make up an overwhelming majority of both victims and offenders of violent crime. Blacks constitute about 12 percent of the U.S. population and Hispanics about 8 percent, but both groups are arrested for a higher proportion of violent crimes. Blacks account for 40 percent of all people arrested for homicides, rapes, armed robberies, and aggravated assaults, and Hispanics account for about 14 percent of people arrested for these violent crimes. For less serious property crimes, blacks are arrested for a quarter to a third of all arsons, car thefts, burglaries, and larceny/thefts; Hispanics are arrested for about 11 percent of these property crimes.

Scholarly efforts to explain these facts have focused on two possibilities. First, race-linked patterns of discrimination, segregation, and concentrated poverty may produce pervasive family and community disadvantages, as well as educational and employment difficulties, which in turn may cause high levels of delinquent and criminal behavior among young minority males. Second is the possibility that, at the hands of the juvenile and criminal justice systems, young black males may be victims of prejudice and discrimination in the form of more frequent arrests, prosecution, and punishment for delinquent and criminal behavior.

Race-linked inequalities may further aggravate problems in many institutional settings in which blacks and whites meet. Because community-level policing practices have at times displayed discriminatory patterns, and because the justice system is nevertheless expected to embody high standards of fairness, justice system interactions have become particularly difficult forums for black-white relations. One result is that many minority inner-city adolescents grow up in environments that, in addition to other difficulties, are characterized by hostility toward the justice system.

## REPORTS REFERENCED

- *Adolescent Behavior and Health* (1978)
- *America's Fathers and Public Policy* (1994)
- *Losing Generations: Adolescents in High-Risk Settings* (1993)
- *New Findings on Poverty and Child Health and Nutrition* (1998)
- *Reducing Risks for Mental Disorders: Frontiers for Preventive Intervention Research* (1994)
- *Schools and Health: Our Nation's Investment* (1997)
- *Youth Development and Neighborhood Influences: Challenges and Opportunities* (1996)

# 4

# Addressing Challenges and Promoting the Healthy Development of Adolescents

There is an interesting contradiction with respect to adolescent health. While adolescence is one of the healthiest periods in the life span—characterized by relatively low incidence of disabling or chronic illnesses, low rates of morbidity and mortality associated with illness or disease, fewer short-term hospital stays, and fewer days away from school because of illness—adolescence is a time when young people are at high risk for engaging in behaviors that can result in poor health outcomes. As mentioned earlier, the U.S. Centers for Disease Control and Prevention has noted that six categories of behavior are responsible for 70 percent of adolescent mortality and morbidity: unintentional and intentional injuries, drug and alcohol abuse, sexually transmitted diseases and unintended pregnancies, diseases associated with tobacco use, illnesses resulting from inadequate physical activity, and health problems due to inadequate dietary patterns.

Fifty years ago, the majority of deaths among adolescents were attributed to natural causes, but there has been a steady decrease in adolescent deaths from cancer, heart disease, and cardiovascular disease. Those declines have been offset in part by steady increases in other leading causes of death and injury. Since the early 1980s, for example, adolescent deaths from homicide, suicide, and the complications of HIV infection have increased. Furthermore, the rates of teenage pregnancy, sexually transmitted diseases, and drug use have either increased or remained at high levels relative to those observed in other countries. Indeed, mortality rates for adolescents have increased since the mid-1980s. Teenage deaths by violence are directly related to economic and social conditions in low-income neighborhoods and to the availability of guns in American society. The rise in teenage homicide and suicide also suggests increasingly high levels of hopelessness, grief, and anger among adolescents. Because of high injury and violence rates, young people in the United States are far more likely to die during adolescence than teenagers in other industrialized countries. Perhaps most important is the fact that the most salient causes of adolescent mortality and morbidity are entirely preventable.

Adolescence is characterized by exploration and experimentation, behaviors that to some extent are developmentally appropriate and socially adaptive, even if they involve a certain amount of risk-taking. Risk-taking involves, among other things, exploration, imagination, developing new and more intimate relationships with peers, testing new levels of independence, establishing a new identity, developing values, unleashing creativity, trying on different hats to see what fits. Carried to extremes, however, risky behaviors may impair mental and physical health. And health risks, such as pregnancy and substance use, may be problems not just when they happen; the consequences of these acts can reach far into the future, and their antecedents are very likely to emerge even before adolescence. But just as adolescence is a time when damaging patterns of behavior can begin to take hold, it also represents an excellent opportunity for the formation of healthful practices.

## SEXUAL RISK, UNINTENDED PREGNANCY, AND SEXUALLY TRANSMITTED DISEASES

A large proportion of adolescents in the United States are engaging in sexual activity and at earlier ages than before, often without the knowledge or skills required to protect themselves from unintended pregnancies and infection with sexually transmitted diseases, including HIV. Studies show that by the 12th grade, nearly 70 percent of adolescents have had sexual intercourse, and approximately a quarter of all students have had sex with four or more partners. This puts many adolescents at high risk for unintended pregnancy, increased incidence of sexually transmitted diseases, and a host of emotional problems associated with a lack of preparation for sex.

For teenagers of different ages, at different stages of cognitive and emotional development, and living under different social, economic, and cultural circumstances, choices concerning sexual behavior reflect very different degrees of rational thinking and conscious decision making. A substantial body of research exists on the variety of individual, family, and social factors associated with adolescent sexual activity. Indeed, research suggests that a number of factors are strongly associated with the initiation of sexual activity before marriage. Among the most important of these are individual characteristics, such as puberty and other developmental characteristics, age, race and socioeconomic status, religiousness, intelligence and academic achievement, and dating behavior; family characteristics, such as family background and parental support and controls; and the influence of peer groups. Thus, although there appears to be a strong relationship between pubertal development, hormone levels, and sexual activity, social factors do intervene in determining when and how both boys and girls initiate sexual intercourse, given maturation.

A substantial body of literature emphasizes the importance of parents and other family members. A number of studies have found that the nature of teenagers' relationship with their parents affects their sexual behavior. As previously discussed, there is growing consensus that adolescents with parents who provide guidance, discipline, and close supervision are significantly less likely to engage in the kinds of behaviors that put them at risk for poor health outcomes—unintended pregnancy, infection with sexually transmitted diseases, involvement in antisocial behaviors, use of drugs—and they are more likely to experience success with their peers and at school. There is also a large body of evidence to suggest that if teenage girls have good lines of communication with their mothers and use their mothers as a source of information about birth control, they are significantly more likely to use contraception. This evidence further emphasizes the importance of parents during the adolescent years and the need for connectedness between adolescents and their parents.

Peers are often cited as the single most important factor affecting the initiation of intercourse by adolescents. It appears, however, that peer influence may have been overrated, particularly for males. However, same-gender peers do appear to be a major source of information about sex. Peer pressure can take several forms (e.g., challenges and dares, coercion, social acceptability), and its influence seems to vary among young people of different ages and genders. Because adolescence in general is a period in which children's orientation shifts away from parents toward peers, it seems likely that peer influence varies according to age. As teens get older, peers become more influential. Although existing research is not conclusive, it also seems likely that the relative influence of peers and parents may also vary depending on the issue. For example, parents may be more important in

to delay initiation of sexual intercourse, avoid unwanted intercourse, and effectively negotiate "safe sex" practices and effective condom use.

Mass media could also play an important role in helping teens protect themselves by airing messages that discourage them from prematurely engaging in sexual behaviors (i.e., before they are emotionally ready or feel comfortable doing so) and encourage them to protect themselves through condom use. Indeed, comprehensive public health messages regarding sexually transmitted diseases, including HIV infection, sexual abuse, and unintended pregnancy, have already shown promise for reducing these risks among adolescents and young adults. Opinion polls show that most Americans support making information regarding sexually transmitted diseases and contraceptives available in the mass media, including the advertising of condoms on television.

For their part, television networks have traditionally banned advertisements for contraceptives until very recently. Condom advertisements on television have been controversial ever since the first such advertisement in 1975. It was not until 1986 that the word "condom" was first used on prime-time television. Recently, the U.S. Centers for Disease Control and Prevention had to fight to use the word "condom" in its public service announcements on HIV prevention. Despite agreeing to air recent announcements about HIV prevention promoting condoms, the networks have restricted the messages to non-prime-time hours. Primarily as a result of the HIV epidemic, in 1991 the Fox Broadcasting Company became the first national television network to run a condom commercial, and some network-owned stations recently have begun to accept condom advertisements, with certain restrictions and so long as they are in "good taste." Some networks, such as Fox and MTV, have been less restrictive in accepting condom advertisements.

Condom use has increased in the past decade, reaching especially high levels among adolescents in part because of these advertisements. Other factors likely to have influenced adolescents' use of condoms include school-based education campaigns and community-based outreach programs. However, condom use tends to decrease as men get older. Although the measures are not completely comparable across the two datasets used, there is clearly a negative association between condom use and age. Even among adolescents ages 15 to 19, there appears to be a decrease in condom use by age, reflecting movement to female methods after initial sexual experiences, during which condoms are often used. One study reports that 16-year-old males who are sexually active use condoms more than 19-year-olds.

Condom use also varies by racial and ethnic affiliation. Black men are the most likely to report using condoms at all ages. Among adolescents, black males use condoms at higher rates than either Hispanic or white males. Although condom use among black adolescent males is higher at last intercourse than among white adolescents, condom use at first intercourse is lower. Since black males, on average, initiate sex about one year earlier than white males, and since earlier ages of first intercourse are associated with less use of contraception, some of the racial difference in condom use at first intercourse is attributable to differences in age at initiation. However, after age at initiation is controlled along with other confounding variables, being a young black man continues to be associated with lower condom use at first intercourse.

Adolescents may face particular barriers in obtaining the more effective methods of contraception. Circumstances vary under which family planning providers will make services available to adolescents, especially if there is no parental involvement. One federal program was designed in part to increase access to contraception among adolescents, but the limited financing and reach of the program means that barriers to access continue to exist for this age group in some circumstances.

Of the many risks associated with early sexual activity, unintended pregnancy and infection with sexually transmitted diseases is perhaps the most widespread. Numerous studies of adolescents have clearly shown that many also have very limited and often faulty information about when fertility begins, the timing of fertility within the menstrual cycle, and the probability of conception. Such misinformation can lead to poor contraceptive use and therefore unintended pregnancy and sexually transmitted diseases.

The proportion of births to unmarried women, including adolescent females, continues to rise. These birth rates, which had declined steadily since World War II, began rising again in 1985, and by 1989 were higher than they had been since the early 1970s. Births to unmarried women represented 15 percent of all births to adolescents in 1960 and 30 percent in 1970; in 1989 over 67 percent of teenage mothers were unmarried, including 92 percent of black teenage mothers.

Because teenage mothers tend to be economically disadvantaged prior to giving birth, it has been difficult to disentangle the consequences of giving birth as a teenager from those of prior disadvantage. Consequences fall both on the young mothers themselves, and on their children. There is evidence to suggest that children of adolescents are at high risk for a wide range of poor outcomes, including health, developmental, and academic problems. As adolescents, children of adolescent mothers are far more likely than those of older mothers to do poorly in school and to engage in high-risk behaviors, including early sexual intercourse and adolescent pregnancy.

Cultural differences may influence the ways that young parents respond to the responsibilities of childrearing: for example, white mothers appear more likely to marry to legitimize their child; blacks are more likely to incorporate the mother and her infant into an extended household, with other adults—usually the adolescent's mother or maternal grandmother or both—assisting with child care. Living with other adults appears to benefit adolescent mothers, who are more likely to complete high school and be employed than those who marry and live in a separate household. Among adolescent mothers receiving Aid to Families with Dependent Children (prior to 1996), blacks were more likely than whites to remain in their parents' home after giving birth, continuing schooling, and delaying marriage; they stayed longer on welfare but were more likely to graduate from high school.

Although much public attention has been given to the growing number of births to unmarried women and to teenage pregnancies, it is only recently that attention has focused on adolescent fathers. Teenage fathers are more likely to come from an economically disadvantaged family and to have completed fewer years of schooling than their childless peers. Although teenage fathers earn more money than their childless counterparts up to age 20, by age 29, those who deferred fatherhood earn roughly 74 percent more than teenage fathers. Teenage fathers are also more likely than their childless peers to commit and be convicted of illegal activity, and their offenses are of a more serious nature. Given their low educational attainment and low earnings, it is not surprising that absent teenage fathers are less likely to pay child support than those who father children in their 20s.

Few men who father children outside marriage subsequently marry the mothers of those children and live with them. But not living in the same household does not necessarily mean lack of involvement with their children. As reported in one study, nearly 80 percent of unmarried fathers who lived near their children visited them every day or several times a week. Ethnographic work also suggests that inner-city young black males usually acknowledged their paternity and that the community supported the young father's participation in informal child support arrangements.

It is often the case that teenage fathers want to spend time with their children, and there is good reason to believe that it is in the best interest of the mother and child to have the father involved. When fathers spend time with their children, research has found them as nurturing as mothers, but in slightly different ways. For example, fathers engaged in more physical play with their children than do mothers. Thus, fathers appear to make a significant and perhaps unique contribution to children's emotional and social development.

A number of programs aimed at encouraging the involvement of young fathers with their children have been developed in recent years. Some of these programs are aimed primarily at improving the educational, parenting, and job skills of young fathers to allow them to better support and interact with their children. Some programs try to capitalize on the desire for involvement, dealing with individual responsibility and self-improvement rather than job training. Few programs, however, have been rigorously evaluated.

## TOBACCO, ALCOHOL, AND ILLICIT DRUGS

Cigarette smoking is the leading cause of avoidable death in the United States. Most smokers begin smoking during childhood and adolescence, with nicotine addiction beginning during the first few years of tobacco use. Decades of research show that, if people do not begin to use tobacco as youngsters, they are highly unlikely to initiate use as adults. Minors consume at least 516 million packs of cigarettes per year, and at least half of those are sold to them illegally. The average age of beginning smoking is 14.5 years; the average age when people become a daily smoker is 17.7 years; of those who have ever smoked daily, 71 percent have done so by age 18.

Many young people are erroneously led to believe that tobacco consumption is widespread among adults, is a social norm among attractive people, and is widespread among vital, successful people who seek to express their individuality, enjoy life, and are socially secure. This message is driven home to children and adolescents by their near-constant exposure to pro-tobacco messages and images (e.g., neighborhood billboards). They also attend cultural and sporting events either sponsored by the tobacco industry or where tobacco logos are prominently displayed.

Research has begun to document the fact that adolescents have a heightened sensitivity to image advertising and promotion, since they are often struggling to define their own identities. Cigarette advertisements are often evocative, play off teenage anxieties, and are positioned to appeal to specific groups defined by social class and ethnic identity. Early adolescence (ages 10 to 14) in particular may be a time of increased susceptibility to the appeal of advertising that promotes certain images attractive to young teenagers.

Clearly, adolescents who choose to use tobacco perceive greater benefits relative to risks. What is most striking, however, is the nature of the trade-off. When children and adolescents begin to use tobacco, they tend to do so for reasons that are transient in nature and closely linked to specific developmental tasks—for example, to assert independence and achieve perceived adult status, or to identify with and establish social bonds with peers who use tobacco. Adolescents who smoke tend to be heavily influenced by their perception of potential social benefits.

With regard to alcohol use, young people of junior high school age drink to a greater extent than was true a generation ago: a larger percentage of them drink, they have their first drinking experience earlier, they drink larger quantities, and they report more frequent intoxication. Furthermore, the generational shift is greater for adolescent girls than for adolescent boys; although girls still do, by and large, drink less than boys, the percentage who drink and who report intoxication experiences has increased more rapidly for girls than for boys.

Marijuana use is often referred to as a gateway drug to other illicit drug use—i.e., other than alcohol, it is often the drug used first, before other drugs such as cocaine, amphetamines, hallucinogenics, and heroin. Throughout the 1980s, national surveys of high school seniors reported a dramatic decline in marijuana use and a general decline in use of other illicit drugs. However, there was a reversal in this trend in the 1990s, particularly among younger students, for the use of various types of illicit drugs, marijuana being most notable.

Adolescents who use alcohol and other drugs recreationally are at greater risk for developing significant health problems resulting from abuse and dependence. Although the patterns, prevalence, and consequences of alcohol, tobacco, and illicit drug abuse in youth populations are not fully understood, a number of individual personality characteristics have been found to be associated with the onset of drinking and illicit drug use among adolescents. They include positive attitudes toward alcohol and other drug use, rebelliousness, tolerance of deviant behavior, low school achievement, lower expectations about academic achievement, and greater opposition to authority. It has also been found that alcohol and other drug abuse and mental health problems often occur simultaneously. Mental health problems that have been found to be associated with increased risk of alcohol and other drug abuse include conduct disorders, attention deficit disorder, and anxiety disorders, particularly phobias and depression. Research has also shown a high degree of overlap between disruptive behavior and drug use in older adolescents, particularly those with a cooccurring conduct disorder.

A number of family factors have also been found to be associated with drug use and abuse among adolescents, including poor quality of the child-parent relationship, family disruption (e.g., divorce and acute or chronic stress), poor parenting, parent or sibling drug use, parental attitudes that are sympathetic to drug use, and neglect.

The peer environment can also make a substantial contribution to alcohol and other drug use. Among older adolescents, peers have a greater effect than parents on alcohol and other drug use and abuse. Typically, adolescent alcohol and other drug use takes place in the company of peers. Peer influence on drug use and abuse may occur in a mutually reinforcing pattern based on the tendency for drug-using adolescents to select similar peers. Studies have not yet demonstrated, however, the influence of peers in the transition from experimental use of alcohol and other drugs to actual abuse (i.e., increased frequency of use, sustained use, and symptoms associated with tolerance and withdrawal).

The sociocultural factors that can have an impact on drug use or abuse include community patterns of drug use. Living in a community with high rates of crime, ready availability of drugs, association with delinquent peers, and acceptance of drug use and abuse are all associated with drug abuse. The larger sociocultural environment also plays a part: alcohol, tobacco, and illicit drugs are frequently reported by news media as having been used by sports and entertainment figures. In addition, social and legal policies (taxes, restrictions on conditions of purchase and use, legal status, and enforcement) can have important effects on access to substances, and consequently abuse.

Ethnographic research designed to explore various risk factors for drug use and abuse, as well as the impact of drug abuse on the community, suggests that the degree of acculturation and assimilation of individuals who are recent immigrants to the United States has been found to be of some importance as a contextual factor, particularly among Mexican Americans. Specifically, children in families who have recently immigrated to the United States or who are first-generation immigrants are at significantly less risk for a wide range of problems, including alcohol, tobacco, and drug use, compared with children in families who are second- and third-generation immigrants. Children in families who are second- and third-generation immigrants—i.e., more assimilated and acculturated—are in turn more likely to resemble U.S.-born children.

In many communities of color, individuals may lack access to broader educational, employment, and consequently economic opportunities, which may also be associated with alcohol and other drug use and abuse. For example, white adolescents typically stop using drugs in their mid-20s, when adult roles of employment and marriage are adopted. In contrast, a significant proportion of black young adults continue drug use well into their adulthood and consequently develop substance abuse disorders.

In American Indian communities, unemployment rates are high, resulting in circumstances in which drug use can flourish. Research has shown that alcoholism is a particular health problem on American Indian reservations. Among American Indian adolescents, school failure and high dropout rates are a serious problem. Also, delinquency and crime are strongly linked to drug use, and gang activity is on the rise among adolescents living on reservations.

Nevertheless, environment—such as communities and neighborhoods—can reinforce a protective sense of self-worth, identity, safety, and environmental mastery. These environmental factors may also serve to protect individuals from drug use and abuse.

Currently more is known about the initiation of drug use than about the transition from use to abuse and dependence. It is clear, however, that adolescents are also vulnerable to the consequences of drug abuse, including health effects, accidents and injuries, violence resulting from illegal activities, and HIV transmission. Adolescent drug abusers differ from adult drug abusers in several ways that are significant for treatment. Of course, adolescent abusers usually have a shorter history of drug abuse; have less severe symptoms of tolerance, craving, and withdrawal; and usually do not have the long-term physical effects of drug abuse. They are, however, at great risk for developing lifelong patterns of drug abuse, which could in turn result in a constellation of negative physical, psychological, and social consequences.

Moreover, the state of knowledge about adolescent treatment is, at best, incomplete. The number of useful studies on adolescents is small, and most of the work that has been conducted in this area is based on studies of treatment outcomes with adults. There are major obstacles to the treatment research with adolescents, such as inconsistent terminology used to refer to adolescent treatment approaches and service components, the use of adult treatment modalities with adolescents, the lack of health care benefits or coverage for alcohol or drug treatment, and a requirement to obtain parental consent for treatment services.

## REPORTS REFERENCED

- *Adolescent Behavior and Health* (1978)
- *AIDS and Behavior: An Integrated Approach* (1994)
- *Assessing the Social and Behavioral Science Base for HIV/AIDS Prevention and Intervention* (1995)
- *The Best Intentions: Unintended Pregnancy and the Well-Being of Children and Families* (1995)
- *Broadening the Base of Treatment for Alcohol Problems* (1990)
- *Dispelling the Myths About Addiction: Strategies to Increase Understanding and Strengthen Research* (1997)
- *Growing Up Tobacco Free: Preventing Nicotine Addiction in Children and Youth* (1994)
- *The Hidden Epidemic: Confronting Sexually Transmitted Diseases* (1997)
- *Improving Health in the Community: A Role for Performance Monitoring* (1997)
- *In Her Own Right: The Institute of Medicine's Guide to Women's Health Issues* (1997)
- *Losing Generations: Adolescents in High-Risk Settings* (1993)
- *New Findings on Poverty and Child Health and Nutrition* (1998)
- *Preventing Drug Abuse: What Do We Know?* (1993)
- *Reducing Risks for Mental Disorders: Frontiers for Preventive Intervention Research* (1994)
- *Research on Mental Illness and Addictive Disorders: Progress and Prospects* (1984)
- *Schools and Health: Our Nation's Investment* (1997)
- *Social Marketing to Adolescent and Minority Populations: Workshop Summary* (1995)
- *Taking Action to Reduce Tobacco Use* (1998)
- *Treating Drug Problems: A Study of the Evolution, Effectiveness, and Financing of Public and Private Drug Treatment Systems* (1990)
- *Violence in Urban America: Mobilizing a Response* (1994)

# 5

# Adolescents Taking Their Place in the World

## ADOLESCENTS IN THE WORKFORCE

In general, the U.S. public believes that work is beneficial—and at worst, benign—for children and adolescents. Today, work is a familiar part of the lives of many children and most adolescents in the United States. Yet working can be dangerous.

The U.S. Department of Labor estimates that about 44 percent of 16- and 17-year-olds work at some time during the year, either while in school, during the summer, or both. The government estimates do not include children younger than 16 who may work, although the National Longitudinal Study of Adolescent Health (called Add Health) found that about 40 percent of 7th and 8th graders were employed during the school year. Children of any age may work in family-owned businesses and on family farms. But even the official numbers for 16- and 17-year-olds are likely to be underestimates because they are based on reports by parents or other adults in the household. Research has found that parents systematically understate the involvement in the workforce of their children. Department of Labor estimates are also limited by rather specific definitions of work. When high school students are interviewed directly through research surveys, about 80 percent report that they hold jobs during the school year at some point during high school.

A notable characteristic of working adolescents is that they move in and out of the labor market, changing jobs and work schedules frequently, in response to changes in employers' needs, labor market conditions, and circumstances in their own lives. Children and teens, like adults, work mainly for the money. Children's income, however, no longer goes primarily toward family support, as it once did: the majority of working adolescents spend most of their incomes on discretionary items or on their individual needs.

The biggest employer of adolescents is the retail sector—restaurants, fast-food outlets, grocery stores, and other retail stores—which employs more than 50 percent of all working 15- to 17-year-olds. The next biggest employer is the service sector (e.g., health care settings such as nursing homes), which accounts for more than 25 percent of working adolescents, followed by 8 percent employed in agriculture. Several of the industries in these sectors of the economy have high rates of injury for all workers.

Some parts of the youth population face unique problems related to work. Children and adolescents who are poor or minority or have disabilities are far less likely than white, middle-class young people to be employed and therefore to reap the potential benefits of work experience. Furthermore, the jobs that poor and minority young people have tend to be in more dangerous industries. When they do work, the hours they work and the wages they receive are comparable to those of other youngsters.

Working has been shown to be associated with both positive and negative consequences for adolescents. Working may increase responsibility, self-esteem, and independence and may help children and adolescents learn valuable work skills. Employment that is limited in intensity (usually defined as 20 hours or less per week) during high school years has been found to promote postsecondary educational attainment. Many studies show positive links between working during high school and subsequent vocational outcomes, including less unemployment, a longer duration of employment after completing schooling, and higher earnings.

However, high-intensity work (usually defined as more than 20 hours per week) is associated with unhealthy and problem behaviors, including substance abuse and minor deviance, insufficient sleep and exercise, and limited time spent with families. Moreover, a high level of work during adolescence has been found to be associated with decreased eventual educational attainment. It should be noted that researchers have often chosen the dividing point of 20 hours of work per week as a convenient way to subdivide hours of work into low-intensity and high-intensity employment; that division is not based on specific research about 20 hours per se.

Children and adolescents may be exposed to many work-related hazards that can result in injury, illness, or death. About 100,000 young people seek treatment in hospital emergency departments for work-related injuries each year. The average of 70 documented deaths that occur among children and adolescents each year as a result of injuries suffered at work is believed to be an underestimate.

The rate of injury per hour worked appears almost twice as high for children and adolescents as for adults—about 4.9 injured per 100 full-time-equivalent workers among adolescents, compared with 2.8 per 100 full-time-equivalent workers for all workers. The industries with the highest injury rates for young workers are retail stores and restaurants, manufacturing, construction, and public-sector jobs. There is virtually no information on the extent to which young people are exposed to toxic or carcinogenic substances in the workplace, exposures that may cause illnesses many years later.

Work-related deaths of workers 17 years and younger are highest in agriculture, followed by retail trade and construction. The most common causes of work-related deaths among 16- and 17-year-olds involve motor vehicles, electrocutions, and homicides.

Many of the industries that employ large numbers of children and adolescents have higher than average injury rates for workers of all ages, but young workers do not receive adequate health and safety training at work—training that has been linked with reduced injuries and acute illnesses when provided to adult workers who are young or inexperienced. Furthermore, children and adolescents often work with inadequate supervision and at tasks for which they may be developmentally unprepared.

Inexperience, as well as physical, cognitive, and emotional developmental characteristics, may also play a part in the risk of injury faced by young workers. Research on adults reveals that inexperience on the job contributes to occupational injuries. It should not be surprising, then, if the inexperience of children and adolescents turns out to be an important factor in their work-related injury rates. Injury may also result from a physical mismatch between the size of the child or adolescent and the task: for example, machinery that was designed for adult males may be too large or heavy for children or adolescents to handle safely.

Working provides benefits to children and adolescents, but the benefits do not come without potential risks to the workers' physical, emotional, educational, and social development. Because so many children and adolescents participate in the U.S. workforce and undoubtedly will continue to do so, the issue is not whether they should work, but what circumstances cause working to be detrimental, what can be done to avoid those circumstances, and how working can be made more beneficial.

## SCHOOL-TO-WORK PROGRAMS

About half of high school graduates in the United States do not go on to college, and of those who do, less than a quarter obtain four-year degrees. Yet the array of programs and services available to college-bound students completely swamps those available to noncollege-bound students. Most students planning to attend college receive comprehensive academic offerings that are linked to college requirements; counseling is available to help them make decisions and to see the connection between academic achievement and college acceptance; once accepted into college, financial assistance is often available; and most institutions offer a variety of orientation services to help adolescents adjust to their new life.

For the larger number of adolescents who do not attend or finish college, assistance is far more limited. Many vocational education and employment training programs do not offer a sequenced series of courses through high school to develop the skills required in specific occupational sectors. The failure of the school-to-work transition system to adequately respond to the needs of the majority of high school graduates contributes materially to the economic insecurity that characterizes many young families.

Traditionally, helping adolescents make the transition into the labor market has not been an explicit part of the mission of America's public schools. As a result, vocational education remains isolated from both academic institutions and the labor market; it is seen as having little value among school administrators and teachers, many of whom argue that vocational education has become a dumping ground for students not in college. The extent of the stigma is disputed, but there is little disagreement that vocational education and its administrators, teachers, and students have become isolated from the mainstream of secondary education, and that recent reforms have done little to reduce this isolation.

For these reasons, vocational education has had at best mixed success. There is abundant evidence that the vocational education system in the United States has only marginally helped students make the transition from schooling to work. In too many vocational programs, there is only a tenuous connection between training and placement, there is no increase in earnings after program completion to offset the cost of training, and few participants find employment appropriate to their training. Vocational students seldom accrue long-term benefits, compared with other students, in terms of income, employment, or job status.

For students in vocational and traditional high school settings, there is no institutional bridge or system to help them make the transition from school to work—unlike in most other industrialized countries. Left to themselves, many high school graduates flounder in the labor market, either jobless or obtaining jobs with low wages and little opportunity for advancement. These difficulties are illustrated by the labor market "inactivity rates" of young people—the percentage of the population that is not employed, serving in the military, or enrolled in school (employment-to-population ratios). For young adults who have failed to graduate from high school, the opportunities for full-time work have been extremely limited.

In the absence of federal policy guidance, there have been a number of state and local efforts to create school-to-work transition systems, with an integrated array of services for young people. School and work linkages have been established through cooperative education, apprenticeship, and other work-based learning programs. There are also a small number of multisite research and demonstration programs—typically funded by foundations—that seek to involve both public and private agencies to provide options for low-achieving students and dropouts to move into the labor market. However, only an estimated 3 to 8 percent of all high school students are enrolled in such programs.

## ADOLESCENTS IN THE 21ST CENTURY: CHANGING SOCIODEMOGRAPHIC PATTERNS

As previously discussed, the size, age, and racial and ethnic composition of the adolescent population is changing dramatically as the 21st century approaches. Added to the growth in the number of adolescents is a tremendous shift currently taking place in the racial and ethnic composition of the nation. The United States is in the midst of a great wave of immigration, a movement of people that has profound implications for a society that by tradition pays homage to its immigrant roots at the same time that it confronts complex and deeply ingrained ethnic and racial divisions. Demographers expect that, by the year 2000, 31 percent of the adolescent population will be members of a racial or ethnic minority group, compared with 26 percent in the total population.

The immigrants of today are coming primarily from nonindustrialized parts of Asia and Latin America and are driving a demographic shift so rapid that, within the lifetimes of today's teenagers, no single ethnic group—including whites of European descent—will constitute a majority of the nation's population.

The demographic shifts are smudging the old lines demarcating two historical, often distinct societies, one black and one white. Reshaped by three decades of rapidly rising immigration, the national portrait is now far more complex. Whites currently account for 74 percent of the children, blacks 12 percent, Hispanics 10 percent, and Asians 3 percent. Yet according to data and predictions generated by the Census Bureau, the population of Hispanics is likely to surpass that of blacks early in the next century. And by the year 2050, it is estimated that Hispanics will account for 25 percent of the population; blacks, 14 percent; Asians, 8 percent; and whites, 53 percent.

Overall, minority groups are growing at a faster rate than the white segments of the population. And these population patterns are particularly apparent when looking at the adolescent population. By the year 2000, the total number of black adolescents is expected to increase 16 percent from 1985; the greatest increase will occur in the younger age group (i.e., 10- to 14-year-olds). Although the absolute number of black adolescents has increased since the mid-1980s, their rates of growth have been smaller than those of Hispanic and Asian adolescents. Thus, although blacks continue to be the largest group among the adolescent minority population, their overall proportion will have decreased from 55 percent in 1985 to 52 percent in 2000.

Projections also indicate that the white adolescent population will have increased by 1 percent between 1985 and 2000. The most dramatic change will be among Hispanic adolescents, with a 42 percent increase in their overall numbers. Hispanic adolescents are expected to represent an estimated 12 percent of the adolescent population. The growth among Hispanics reflects both an increasing number of new immigrants and improvements in the manner in which Hispanics are counted in the population. In addition, as a result of Asian migration, demographers also estimate that, in the year 2000, 11 percent of all school-age children will be of Asian or Pacific Island descent.

From the standpoint of adolescent development, it is difficult to draw firm conclusions about similarities and differences between adolescents in immigrant and U.S.-born families regarding psychological well-being, academic success, and other measures of successful adaptation to U.S. society, for reasons that include the small immigrant samples used in available studies. However, the majority of adolescents in immigrant families appear to sustain positive feelings about themselves and their well-being, while also perceiving that they have relatively less control over their lives and are less popular with their peers at school. Many also report having strong achievement motivation, although this may deteriorate from one generation to the next.

Children in immigrant families also appear to have somewhat higher middle school grade point averages and math test scores than do children in U.S.-born families, although reading test scores for the first generation are lower than for later generations. Differences across children and adolescents from various countries of origin appear quite large, however. For example, Chinese adolescents in immigrant families have higher grade point averages and higher math test scores than Chinese-origin or white children in U.S.-born families. In contrast, Mexican-origin children in immigrant and U.S.-born families have grade point averages and math test scores that are similar to each other but much lower than for white children in U.S.-born families. Corresponding to the declines in achievement motivation across generations, there is evidence among Chinese and Filipino children that the especially strong achievement records of the second generation are not sustained in later generations.

Demographic change, worldwide and within the United States, will powerfully affect many aspects of the quality of life for adolescents in the 21st century—the environment, food, the economy, schools, jobs, and health. America's health care system in the 21st century must successfully achieve equity between the young and the aged and among social and ethnic groups.

Given these dramatic demographic shifts and the substantial increase in the adolescent population in the coming years, researchers have the opportunity to increase their knowledge base with regard to promoting adolescent development, health, safety, security and well-being; designing and, in some cases, redesigning institutions and systems of care to more appropriately address the needs of adolescents; promoting peaceful, respectful relations among adolescents of different ethnic groups; promoting positive relationships between adolescents and their parents; encouraging and supporting them as a resource within communities; and helping them define their civic role in a democratic society.

## REPORTS REFERENCED

- *America's Children:  Health Insurance and Access to Care* (1998)
- *From Generation to Generation: The Health and Well-Being of Children in Immigrant Families* (1998)
- *Losing Generations: Adolescents in High-Risk Settings* (1993)
- *The New Americans: Economic, Demographic, and Fiscal Effects of Immigration* (1997)
- *New Findings on Welfare and Children's Development: Summary of a Research Briefing* (1994)
- *Protecting Youth at Work: Health, Safety, and Development of Working Children and Adolescents in the United States* (1999)
- *Systems of Accountability: Implementing Children's Health Insurance Programs* (1998)
- *Transitions in Work and Learning: Implications for Assessment* (1997)
- *2020 Vision: Health in the 21st Century* (1996)

# 6

# Implications for Research and Linking Research to Policy and Practice

Although research and new policies and programmatic initiatives have documented the many problems that adolescents face in an increasingly complex and diversified society, a clear federal policy mandate is lacking that sets forth funding and policy priorities, and that could provide guidance for how to approach the needs of diverse adolescent populations (Brindis et al., 1998). The complexity of those needs, and the ambivalence expressed by society concerning the role of adolescents, have made it difficult to establish a focused agenda for youth-related issues. Progress in the coming decade requires that the field take a step back, map out the areas in which additional research is needed, identify opportunities for research to inform policy and practice, and proceed in a thoughtful and coordinated manner to address these needs.

In this chapter we outline a number of issues that will become increasingly important and that the Forum on Adolescence expects to explore. These include the implications of a changing adolescent population; new research methodologies and approaches needed to further advance understanding of adolescent health and development; strategies to strengthen and support relationships between teenagers and their parents; the continued development of indicators of adolescent well-being; approaches to integrating frameworks for preventing risk behaviors and promoting positive developmental outcomes among youth; the delivery of developmentally appropriate health care services to youth; and ensuring adolescents' safe and productive use of new technologies.

## INCREASING NUMBERS AND GROWING DIVERSITY

As discussed earlier in this report, the size and composition of the adolescent population is expected to change dramatically during the coming decades—i.e., there will be more adolescents than ever before. Moreover, white teenagers will no longer be the majority group, and Hispanic teenagers will outnumber black teenagers. Now is the time to ask if current systems and policies are prepared to respond to these changes. Are private and public institutions and systems (e.g., education, employment, housing, transportation, and health) prepared to respond to these trends? How will institutions and systems need to be redesigned to respond appropriately? How can a national youth policy agenda be developed to ensure the health and well-being of this segment of the population?

With this increase in diversity, coupled with worldwide patterns of increased mobility and migration, cooperative relations among different racial and ethnic groups are essential to the nation's future. Yet there is growing evidence to suggest that white youth and youth from ethnic minority groups hold deeply divergent views on how to relate to each other. The harmful results of this racial divide among youth are becoming more apparent as demonstrated by an alarming increase of adolescent hate crimes, organized hate groups, and overt expressions of racial intolerance.

Research is needed to characterize how youth derive a sense of belonging and personal meaning from their ethnic and other affiliations, as well as on how youth understand, interpret, and experience such constructs as race, ethnicity, racism, and all other forms of discrimination. While there is growing evidence that strategies can be crafted to create positive intergroup relations, there is little agreement regarding what intervention strategies are essential to promote peaceful, respectful relations or to prevent conflict and violence among youth stemming from ethnic identity. Certainly, ethnicity is not the only defining characteristic of teenagers. They also differ from one another according to their physical, cognitive, and learning abilities; body shape and size; religious and political beliefs and values; sexual orientation; and interests and expressions of creativity. Future efforts are needed to encourage and support enduring changes in the ways that teenagers relate and interact with their peers who are different from themselves. As a society, the goal should be to help young people promote peaceful, respectful relations among all youth.

## HEALTHY ADOLESCENT DEVELOPMENT

The study of adolescence is becoming an increasingly sophisticated science. Thanks to powerful new research tools and other scientific and technological advances, today's theories of adolescent development are more likely to be supported by scientific evidence than in the past. Indeed, there has been sufficient research to allow a reassessment of the nature of adolescent development. At the same time, there is greater recognition that neither puberty nor adolescence can be understood without considering the social, psychological, and cultural contexts in which young people grow and develop, including the familial and societal values, social and economic conditions, and institutions that they experience. In the past, researchers tended to conduct research designed to examine the impact of hormones on adolescent behavior. While this work continues, there is now an appreciation for the complex reciprocal relationship and interaction between biological, psychological, and social environments and the interaction between these environments and adolescent behavior.

The field of adolescence is also increasingly benefiting from the fact that researchers from diverse fields, including the biological, behavioral, and social sciences, have developed new techniques to study adolescent development. Use of more rigorous research methods has improved the reliability and validity of the measurement techniques used, and consequently the ability to document the multifaceted dimensions of growth and maturation during adolescence.

For example, the development of radioimmunoassay methodology in the late 1960s, and the considerable refinement of that process over the decades, have made it possible to study the hormones that control reproductive maturation. The development of neuroimaging technology in the 1970s created exciting new opportunities for studying brain development; these techniques include more sensitive, easy-to-use hormone assay technology and new brain-imaging technologies, allowing insight into brain development and function.

Moreover, longitudinal studies are increasingly being designed to characterize the interaction among genetic, biological, familial, environmental, social, and behavioral factors (both risk and protective in nature) among children and adolescents. For example, a valuable new source of data that has the potential to significantly advance the knowledge base of physiological and behavioral development among adolescents is the National Longitudinal Study of Adolescent Health (Add Health). From the collection of longitudinal data, it will be possible to examine how the timing and tempo of puberty influences social and cognitive development among teenagers. This dataset will also permit analyses to examine how family-, school-, and individual-level risk and protective factors are associated with adolescent health and morbidity (e.g., emotional health, violence, substance use, sexuality).

Despite advances in the science and knowledge base, it remains the case that current understanding of adolescent development is rather limited. The research conducted to date has been predominately descriptive in nature, has relied on cross-sectional data and adolescent self-report and has been unidimensional in focus. Indeed, few research studies have successfully considered the multiple factors that collectively influence adolescent development. There is now a growing appreciation, however, that new research is needed, including research that employs longitudinal designs; characterizes developmental changes associated with the onset of puberty well before the age of 8; and seeks to characterize growth and development across the life span—i.e., from infancy to adolescence, young adulthood, adulthood, and the senior years.

Studying these developmental stages in isolation from one another provides only a partial and incomplete picture. In addition, while the current literature is rich with respect to research that characterizes adolescents' involvement in risk and risk-related behaviors, research on risk factors is only correlational or bidirectional in nature, which tells only half the story. It examines the extent to which, in any given sample of adolescents and at any given time, teens exposed to a risk factor are doing worse in some respect compared with children who are not exposed to that same risk factor. It says nothing about the base rates of either the risk factors or the outcomes. Base rates could be rising or falling, while the correlations between risk factors and outcomes could be quite undisturbed. This means, for example, that although it may not matter greatly whether there are increasing or decreasing numbers of adolescents in poverty; it is also true that those in poverty are still at risk.

Finally, previous research has been limited when it has assumed that adolescents, as a segment of the population, are a homogenous group. We now know that while all adolescents experience the biological, cognitive, and social transitions of this period, not all adolescents experience these changes in the same way. For example, puberty makes some adolescents feel adult-like, attractive, and confident; it makes others feel awkward, unattractive, and self-conscious. Being able to think in abstract and hypothetical terms offers some teenagers the opportunity to imagine the wide range of possibilities that exist for their future; it prompts others to feel uncertainty and despair. While the fundamental changes associated with adolescence are universal, there is wide variation in the ways in which adolescents experience these changes, and this variation is largely accounted for by the child's interpretation of these changes, as well as the environment in which these changes occur. As described by Bronfenbrenner (1979), the psychological impact of the biological, cognitive, and social changes of adolescence is shaped by the environment in which these changes take place. These considerations need to be further explored by research.

## RELATIONSHIPS BETWEEN TEENAGERS AND PARENTS

Adolescence is not just a time of major developmental changes in children; it is also a time of significant transformations and realignment in family relations. Raising adolescents can certainly be stressful and difficult for parents who are likely to feel less adequate and more anxious and stressed than when their children were younger. Raising a teenager can also be rewarding, and families as well as other supportive adults clearly matter with respect to the healthy development of adolescents.

As discussed by Small (1990), there have been a number of recent changes in American society and in the nature of adolescence that have also contributed to the challenge of raising adolescents today:

• The length of time during which adolescents rely on their parents for financial, emotional, and material support is increasing, with more and more young adults in their early 20s living at home or financially dependent on their parents, resulting in a protracted period of responsibility for parents and a greater uncertainty regarding how to raise adolescents.
• Parents have become confused about how best to prepare adolescents for future adult roles as a result of rapid sociocultural change and the multiple and often competing sources of information and values that are increasingly complex in a diverse society.
• Parents are often worried as a result of the greater number of potentially dangerous activities, substances, and influences to which contemporary adolescents are exposed.

Compared with research on families with young children, there has been much less attention to the home and family environments of adolescents. Yet it is clear, as this report discusses, that adolescents develop best when they live and develop in a supportive home and family environment. Despite the fact that adolescents are moving out beyond the family and striving for greater autonomy, parents remain an important influence in the lives of their adolescent children. · In a paper published by Resnick and colleagues, early analyses from the National Longitudinal Study of Adolescent Health found that teenagers who have strong emotional attachments to their parents and teachers are much less likely to use drugs and alcohol, attempt suicide, engage in violence, or become sexually active at an early age (Resnick et al., 1997). The authors concluded that feeling loved, understood, and paid attention to by parents helps teenagers avoid high-risk activities, regardless of whether they come from a one- or a two-parent household. At school, positive relationships with teachers were found to be more important in protecting teenagers than any other factor, including classroom size or the amount of training a teacher has.

What are the practical implications of research on parenting adolescents, and how can research, policy, and practice be linked? Very little is known about how to educate and support parents of adolescents most effectively and enhance their childrearing abilities. There is an enormous gap between what is known about the effects of parenting on adolescents as it naturally occurs and what can be done to enhance it when parents struggle. This gap is especially striking in light of the recent growth in the development and availability of parenting programs, videos, articles, and books aimed at supporting and guiding parents of adolescents. Research on best practices and the effectiveness of education, training, and support programs and materials is almost nonexistent. Understanding of the types of knowledge, skills, and supports that parents of adolescents need and desire, as well as the strategies and change techniques that are likely to be most helpful and effective, is also very limited. Research is therefore needed to further strengthen relationships between teenagers and their parents and to provide support to parents of adolescents.

## NEW TRENDS IN ADOLESCENT BEHAVIOR

The past few years have seen a number of encouraging changes and even reversals in trends in some of the leading causes of mortality and morbidity among adolescents. While these trends are not consistent across all causes of death, problems, or risk behaviors, these data are promising and they do suggest that some combination of events—whether it is new ways in which social services are addressing the needs of adolescents, new approaches to the design and delivery of prevention and health promotion interventions, or new policies—has had a positive impact on the health, safety, and security of teenagers in the United States. The following pages highlight a few of these trends, including recent rates of adolescent mortality, adolescent pregnancy, school dropout, and use of tobacco, alcohol, and other illicit drugs.

### Adolescent Mortality

As discussed in this report, adolescents have much higher mortality rates compared with younger children. In 1980, the death rate among adolescents was 98 per 100,000. This rate then decreased to 89 in 1991, and further declined to 84 in 1995 (see Figure 6-1). Injury, which includes homicide, suicide, and unintentional injuries, continues to account for 4 out of 5 or 78 percent of deaths among adolescents. While accidents continue to account for more than twice as many teen deaths as any other source, including homicide, examination of recent trends in causes of death among teenagers reveals some changes. Between 1985 and 1996, the number of teen deaths due to accidents fell from 8,202 in 1985 to 6,756 in 1996, while the number of teen homicides increased from 1,602 to 2,924 during the same period. However, between 1994 and 1996, the number of

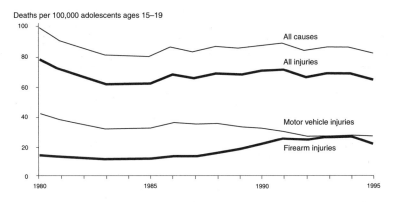

**FIGURE 6-1** Mortality rate among adolescents ages 15 to 19 by cause of death, 1980-1995. SOURCE: Data from Centers for Disease Control and Prevention, National Center for Heath Statistics, National Vital Statistics System.

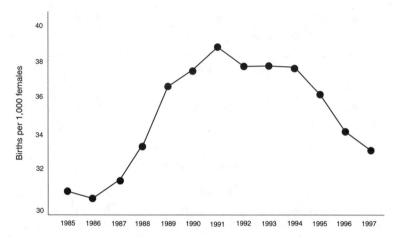

**FIGURE 6-2**   Birth rate of 15- to 17-year-olds: 1985 to 1997. SOURCE: Data from National Center for Health Statistics.

teen homicides fell by 18 percent, which may signal a change in long-term trends. The annual number of teen suicides also decreased, albeit slightly, from 1,849 to 1,817, between 1985 to 1996.

## Adolescent Pregnancy

As previously discussed, teenage childbearing is problematic because it often diminishes the opportunities of both the child and the young mother. Births to females under age 18 are particularly troublesome because most of these mothers are unmarried, and the vast majority have not completed high school. Nationally, the birth rate to teenagers has been decreasing over the past several years. In 1991, the birth rate among 15- to 17-year-olds was 39 per 1,000 females, and between 1991 to 1997, this rate decreased to 33. This rate increased slightly, however, in 1997, to 34 per 1,000 females (see Figure 6-2). The birth rate among 18- to 19-year-olds also declined between 1991 and 1996, and blacks, Hispanics, and whites have all experienced the decline.

## School Dropout

As previously discussed, graduating from high school is critical for obtaining postsecondary education or getting a good job. Indeed, teens who drop out of high school face enormous odds of achieving financial success in life. Nationwide, there was very little change in this measure between 1985 and 1996. In 1985, 11 percent of teens ages 16 to 19 were high school dropouts, compared with 10 percent in 1996. There was, however, a slight decline in the percentage of 16- to 19-year-olds not attending school and not working, from 11 percent in 1985 to 9 percent in 1996.

## Tobacco, Alcohol, and Illicit Drug Use

Alcohol and illicit drug use has both short- and long-term implications with respect to the health and development of adolescents. Long-term trends indicate that heavy drinking, defined as drinking five or more alcoholic beverages in a row in the last two weeks, peaked in 1981 with 41 percent of high school seniors reporting this behavior. The percentage of seniors reporting heavy drinking then declined significantly, to a low of 18 percent in 1993. Unfortunately, since 1993, the prevalence of this behavior has risen to 31 percent. In 1997, almost 1 in 3 12th graders, 1 in 4 10th graders, and more than 1 in 10 8th graders reported heavy drinking (Federal Interagency Forum on Child and Family Statistics, 1997).

According to data reported by the Monitoring the Future study, marijuana, cocaine, and heroin use bottomed out in the early 1990s but has since risen among children at all grade levels (see Figure 6-3) (Backman et al., 1998). However, data for 1997 and 1998 suggest that this trend toward increased illicit drug use is leveling off and may be in the process of reversing. For example, annual use of any illicit drug by high school seniors peaked at 54.2 percent in 1979, declined to a low of 27.1 percent in 1992, then climbed steadily to 42.4 percent in 1997. Annual marijuana use among high school seniors crested in 1979 at 50.8 percent, then declined to 21.9 percent in 1992, before rising steadily to 38.5 percent in 1997. Annual cocaine use more than doubled among high school seniors, from 5.6 percent in 1975 to 13.1 percent in 1985, then decreased to 4.9 percent in 1996. Seniors' use of any illicit drug, marijuana, and cocaine has, however, been stable since 1996.

Unfortunately, these same encouraging trends are not apparent for tobacco use by adolescents. The percentage of 8th, 10th, and 12th graders who reported that they smoked cigarettes daily increased between 1992 and 1997 (Backman et al., 1998). In 1997, 25 percent of 12th graders reported smoking daily during the previous 30 days, as did 18 percent of 10th graders and 9 percent of 8th graders. Prior to 1992,

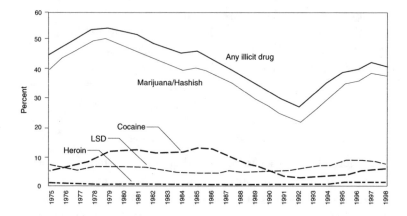

**FIGURE 6-3**    Trends in past-year use of drugs by high school seniors. SOURCE: Adapted by the National Institute on Drug Abuse from data compiled by Backman et al. (1998).

smoking had been decreasing among 12th graders since 1980, when 21 percent of 12th graders reported that they smoked daily (Federal Interagency Forum on Child and Family Statistics, 1997).

## ADOLESCENT WELL-BEING

Because the federal and state governments are organized to identify needs and to address and solve problems, it tends to collect data on problems, such as morbidity, mortality, poverty, and crime. So trends in drug use, violence, and sexual activity are often mentioned, but we rarely hear about the commitment of youth to recycling or to work they do around the house or outside, close parent-child relations, or the time that youth spend volunteering (Moore, 1998). To provide a more balanced perspective, data are needed to assess not only the problems experienced by youth and poor developmental outcomes, but also positive indicators of safety, security, and well-being. This will require the development of new measures and the collection of new data at the federal, state, and local levels. Possible constructs include community involvement, recycling, volunteering, religious practice and activities, exercise and sports, activities in school clubs, civic engagement, reading and participation in cultural affairs, family activities, and work done in the home. The lives of children are complex and multifaceted. Indicators should reflect the complexities of adolescents' lives. For example, long-term poverty is more problematic than short-term spells of poverty, and cumulative risks undermine child development more than a single risk. And average values do not reflect the diversity experienced by children and adolescents from varied backgrounds.

Until very recently, research and services have been largely problem focused, funded by categorical "problem identified" funding streams, and driven by policies that rarely view problems as interrelated. Federal statistics on children and adolescents are similarly highly fragmented and administered by different agencies, each with its own interests and each with distinctive histories and constituencies. This suggests the need for improvements in data collection and reporting systems in order to ascertain the connections between resources and outcomes and also to identify the family and community processes that translate resources into outcomes.

During the past five years, a great deal of scientific and policy-related activity has taken place around the development and use of child and youth indicators (Hauser et al., 1997). In addition, there have been several important attempts to broaden existing conceptual frameworks in order to support more multidisciplinary approaches to the study of child and youth well-being (Brooks-Gunn et al., 1995; Family and Child Well-Being Research Network, 1999). For example, some researchers are now attempting to develop indicators that could provide informative measures of youth's perceptions of their own safety and security and their willingness to invest time and resources in preparing for long-term goals as opposed to short-term advantages. Others are using measures of youth potential and connectedness to examine positive aspects of youth development (such as indicators of personal and family responsibility, civic engagement, and community service) that are often overlooked in datasets focused narrowly on the presence or absence of problem behaviors. At the community level, some scholars are experimenting with measures designed to judge the capacity of a neighborhood or other social setting to support the values of its residents, including youth, in achieving positive social, economic, and personal benefits (see Hauser et al., 1997).

These scientific efforts have been quite successful in pushing the field forward by taking advantage of existing data sources. However, these efforts have uncovered substantial holes in existing models, in available measures of key constructs, and in the contents of longitudinal and cross-sectional surveys. Thus, future research is needed to operationally define indicators of well-being and of safety and security as necessary for assessing and monitoring well-being among youth, including their perceptions of health and well-being. New measurement tools and methodologies that can be used to collect these data are also likely to be needed. Once developed, further work will be needed to integrate these new indicators into the evaluations of interventions intended to promote positive developmental outcomes among youth, and into data systems intended to monitor national, state, and local-level trends in the health and well-being of adolescents.

## PROGRAMS FOR INTERVENTION AND YOUTH DEVELOPMENT

In seeking to explain variations in adolescent development, researchers have focused traditionally on personal characteristics, family relationships, and friendships. Such lines of inquiry suggest that these factors interact across multiple dimensions to influence youth outcomes. Different theories have emerged over the past decade that provide frameworks to guide research and youth service programs, especially in meeting the needs of disadvantaged youth (National Research Council, 1993). Some of these efforts emphasize the role of the individual in terms of biological and psychological interactions that shape youth identity and decision-making processes during adolescence. Others focus on family or peer interactions and the ways in which adolescents negotiate greater autonomy while still needing support during their teenage years.

As discussed in this report, researchers have increasingly focused on the social settings in which youth develop. This has prompted new research inquiry designed to explore how individual, family, and peer relationships and outcomes are influenced by factors such as physical environment, economic opportunity structures, and ethnic and social networks, especially in urban areas characterized by concentrated poverty (see Duncan and Brooks-Gunn, 1997). Scholars are also investigating relationships between types and density of social interactions, youth perceptions of positive and negative influences within their social and physical environments, and ways in which these relationships and perceptions are associated with the emergence of problem behaviors within communities (such as crime, gangs, substance abuse, child maltreatment, and unintended teen pregnancy).

Longitudinal studies and other research now suggest that complex social support interactions occur (or not) as a result of a mix of physical and social factors in community settings that affect youth's perception of their own strengths and deficits, family life, and choice of friends and role models (Carnegie Council on Adolescent Development, 1995).

This research on settings suggests that certain implicit social norms, behaviors, resources, and networks in affluent or higher resource settings that are often taken for granted (such as good schools; recreational and sports programs; safe homes and social centers; private health care; attitudes toward the value of work, education, community service, and parenting; and beliefs about future career and employment opportunities) constitute positive assets that have profound impact on the ways in which youth prepare themselves for their adult lives. Conversely, the absence of these assets creates significant gaps in the social support and opportunity structure for youth as they experience important transitions in becoming adults.

In addition, the presence of individuals and groups who represent sources of danger, insecurity, and deviant role models can diminish youth's motivation in preparing for productive and meaningful relationships and create cynicism about their opportunities to achieve participatory membership in society. Conversely, the presence of individuals who serve as positive role models may give youth a sense of optimism and the belief in future opportunities, as well as discourage them from engaging in risk behaviors. These attitudes and beliefs—whether they are pessimistic or optimistic—influence the types of choices and behaviors that young people acquire during their developmental years.

The influence of settings is also likely to be mediated by the child's mind, i.e., by the child's interpretation and perception of his or her experiences within these settings. For this reason, changing the institutions—neighborhoods and schools—without attending to the adolescent's construction and interpretation of those changes will not have the intended effects on most children.

Scholars from multiple disciplines are presently engaged in developing theory and indicators that relate to the relations between social settings and youth development. Experimental program initiatives are under way to improve teenagers' engagement and involvement with their communities and use of available resources and supports. Unfortunately, researchers often lack the opportunity to interact and work with those who are responsible for designing and implementing youth development programs. Research evaluations of program interventions and their outcomes, in particular, reflect the absence of a shared vision about the overall mission of youth development initiatives and the capacity of a program to achieve ambitious, long-term goals.

Public and private agencies are now increasingly experimenting with a wide array of youth development interventions that are designed to foster social support for youth by two approaches: (1) strengthening the ability of youth to interact successfully with community resources and networks, and (2) improving the capacity of community programs and services to engage youth in their efforts. Such efforts include mentorship programs (such as Big Brothers/Big Sisters); school-based community service efforts (such as volunteer programs); school-to-work transition programs (such as YouthBuild); teen pregnancy, substance abuse, or violence prevention programs; and others (see Dryfoos, 1998). Significantly, rather than focus on the deficits of today's youth (such as delinquency, drug use, teenage pregnancy, and violence), many of these programs focus on the resilience of youth and reconfiguring assets within the community in an effort to promote positive youth developmental outcomes (Blum, 1998).

Although some approaches appear to be promising because of their ability to sustain broad youth-adult relationships, no single approach is yet strong enough to provide general guidance for the field. As a result, program sponsors, service providers, and researchers are examining the reasoning behind different interventions and the outcome measures associated with their use. Program participants are also keenly interested in knowing how the impacts of broader types of youth development initiatives compare with other, more narrowly focused problem prevention interventions such as teen pregnancy, substance abuse, and violence prevention efforts.

Community-based youth programs can provide enriching and rewarding experiences for young adolescents, and many do: their young members socialize with their peers and adults and learn to set and achieve goals, compete fairly, win gracefully, recover from defeat, and resolve disputes peaceably. These programs also provide children and adolescents with the opportunity to acquire life skills—i.e., the ability to communicate effectively, make decisions, solve problems, make plans, and set goals for education and careers.

Considerable work is needed to inform the design, implementation, and evaluation of programs targeted to youth. Clearly, no single program approach will be appropriate for all adolescents: one size does not fit all. The challenge therefore becomes one of designing a range of intervention strategies that are comprehensive and interdisciplinary in nature, that are developmentally appropriate and culturally relevant, and that take advantage of the many settings or environments in which children and adolescents grow and develop—e.g., the home, schools, communities, social services, the media, and the business or corporate sector. Other questions will also need to be addressed. For example, what are programs really trying to accomplish and how can they be designed to accomplish these goals? Conceptually, how are such constructs as safety, security, and well-being defined, and can programs be designed to accomplish this? What are appropriate outcomes and what are the strengths and limitations of existing data sources and data collection instruments? How do we move beyond evaluating programs by measuring the presence or absence of problem behaviors, to measuring the presence or absence of positive developmental outcomes and well-being? How can evaluations look at both short-term or interim effects and long-term outcomes? What is known about the youth who access after-school and community services and those who do not? What are the implications if those who are most vulnerable or in greatest need do not choose to take advantage of these services? Are certainly types of programs more or less effective with specific segments of the population?

Finally, the field needs to consider what are appropriate expectations for these programs in term of individual-level outcomes. For example, it is clearly unrealistic to think that a single three-month community-based after-school program will have such a profound impact that it will overcome competing deficits or problems, such as a dysfunctional home; overcrowded schools with few resources and poorly trained teachers; and impoverished and disorganized communities with few social services.

## DEVELOPMENTALLY APPROPRIATE
## HEALTH CARE SERVICES

During the past decade, the health status of adolescents and young adults has been the subject of growing concern among policy makers, researchers, clinicians, and advocates interested in youth issues and adolescent health. Poor health outcomes caused by health-damaging behaviors, compounded by inadequate use of available health resources, have led to a number of national efforts to study the special health, social, economic, and legal needs of adolescents. An unprecedented number of books examining the health and well-being of youth, as well as a host of federal, state, and foundation reports, has offered an overwhelming array of recommendations for addressing the spectrum of problems experienced by adolescents (Brindis et al., 1998).

The teenage years provide an important window of opportunity to provide youth with guidance and support to avoid behaviors that involve risk and to encourage a healthful lifestyle, including but not limited to exercise, a healthful diet, and healthful sleep patterns. Health care providers can play an important role in this respect. Unfortunately, there are a number of barriers that prevent adolescents from accessing and utilizing primary health, preventive, and specialty services. Barriers to adolescents receiving care include lack of experience in negotiating complex medical systems; reticence in seeking care for potentially embarrassing needs, such as reproductive or mental health concerns; concern about confidentiality and parental consent laws; fragmented care; and distance from medical facilities. However, access to health services, especially for ambulatory care, depends in large part on the ability to pay for services, and adolescents and young adults are less likely to have health insurance than other age groups (Newacheck et al., 1990). Moreover, adolescents who lack health insurance have been found to be in poorer health than those who do have adequate insurance. Clearly efforts are needed to address these barriers and to increase teenagers' access to and use of needed health care and preventive services.

Teenagers with a chronic illness or disability are a segment of the adolescent population that warrants special attention. These youth are defined as having a chronic condition that results in limitations in daily activities that require ongoing services to maintain or enhance daily life function. It is estimated that nearly 2 million adolescents (6 percent) ages 10 to 18 have a chronic condition that limits their daily activities. Within this 6 percent of the adolescent population, the major physical disabilities include chronic respiratory conditions (21 percent) and diseases of the musculoskeletal system (15 percent). Youth with disabilities make greater use of health and hospital services than the rest of the adolescent population.

In many respects, there has been insufficient attention to the needs of children and adolescents with chronic debilitating conditions and with disabilities, and there are a number of very important policy-related questions that can and should be informed by research and analysis of available data. For example, there is considerable debate among policy makers, health care providers, and families with a disabled child about current definitions of disability and criteria or tools for determining disability. Other questions relate to the provision of care, such as what are the patterns of providing care for children with disabilities? What are the effective ways of providing care? How accessible are they? How are existing health insurance and managed care plans covering these services? How are other forms of coverage, such as Medicaid and the new State Children's Health Insurance Program, covering these children? What care is provided by families at reasonable levels of cost and burden? What are appropriate standards for the duration of benefits, such as the factors that can predict the long-term prognosis of children and adolescents with disabilities? What are effective ways to advance such children toward economic independence? What are appropriate incentives to encourage children to develop to their full potential? All of these questions must be addressed in order to help these young people grow and develop to their full potential.

## THE MEDIA AND ADVANCES IN TECHNOLOGY

Adolescents today have greater access to more kinds of media and technology than ever before. In the midst of a world-wide communications explosion, with relatively recent advances in computer and telecommunications technology, adolescents are spending considerable amounts of time online. Indeed, recent advances in media and computer technology, including satellite transmission, remote control, the video cassette recorder, computers, and the Internet, have exponentially expanded the number and kinds of media, and have given teens more control over when and where they use them. Advances in various forms of media and computer technology, including the Internet, has changed the ways in which children and adolescents access information in both their home and their classrooms. Many teenagers now actively communicate through electronic mail with their peers around the world. They share ideas, interests, opinions, and beliefs regarding a wide range of issues and current events. There is also evidence that teenagers are becoming more interested in civic engagement through the Internet, but defined on their terms. However, it is clear that all children and adolescents do not have equal access to these technologies, and it is not clear what the long-term implications will be of these inequities.

Children and adolescents are likely to benefit greatly from the wealth of information and educational materials available on the Internet, as well as valuable skills that are likely to ensure their competitiveness in the workforce. There is also growing concern about children and adolescents' access to information and material that are developmentally inappropriate and even potentially harmful. As a result, there has been a growing interest on behalf of the public and policy makers to identify the range of tools and strategies that can be used to ensure children's safe and appropriate use of the Internet.

The Internet and future technologies will no doubt continue to play an important role in the lives of teenagers worldwide. Research is therefore needed to characterize how children and adolescents use the Internet and what are their experiences with it; what technological and nontechnological tools might be used by parents, educators, librarians, local communities, and state and federal policy makers to ensure children's safe and appropriate use of the Internet; ensure that the Internet is used to its full potential— i.e., to enhance learning opportunities and promote the healthy development of children and adolescents. Finally, research is needed to explore how the various forms of the media and social marketing strategies can be used to encourage or reinforce health-promoting behaviors among adolescents.

## ROLE OF THE FORUM

The forum undertook this report to inform its future work. From the body of research considered for this synthesis, we were impressed by how much is now known about adolescent development, as well as overwhelmed by how much is still unknown about how to ensure the safety, security, and well-being of adolescents. The task for us—and all those in research, policy, and practice—is to extract from this report the most fruitful avenues for the next steps.

# References

Backman, J.G., et al.
>1998 National survey results on drug use. In *Monitoring the Future Study 1975-1997*. Volume I, Secondary School Students. Bethesda, MD: National Institute on Drug Abuse.

Blum, R.W.
>1998 Healthy youth development as a model for youth health promotion: A review. *Journal of Adolescent Health* 22:368-375.

Brooks-Gunn, J., et al.
>1995 *New Social Indicators of Child Well-Being.* The Family and Child Well-Being Network. Vienna, Austria: European Centre for Social Welfare Policy and Research.

Brindis, C.D., et al.
>1998 *Improving Adolescent Health: An Analysis and Synthesis of Health Policy Recommendations.* Full Report. San Francisco: National Adolescent Health Information Center, University of California, San Francisco.

Brofenbrenner, U.
>1979 *The Ecology of Human Development.* Cambridge, MA: Harvard University Press.

Bureau of the Census
>1965 Estimates of the population of the United States by single years of age, color, and sex: 1900 to 1959. *Current Population Reports* Series P-25, No. 311. Washington, D.C.: U.S. Department of Commerce.

>1974 Estimates of the population of the United States by age, sex, and race: April 1, 1960 to July 1, 1973. *Current Population Reports* Series P-25, No. 519. Washington, D.C.: U.S. Department of Commerce.

>1982 Preliminary estimates of the population of the United States by age, sex, and race: 1970 to 1981. *Current Population Reports* Series P-25, No. 917. Washington, D.C.: U.S. Department of Commerce.

1996   Population projections of the United States by age, sex, and race and Hispanic origin: 1995 to 2050. *Current Population Reports* Series P-25, No. 1130. Washington, D.C.: U.S. Department of Commerce.

1999   Unpublished estimate tables for 1980 to 1997. U.S. Bureau of the Census web site. Available electronically: www.census.gov.

Carnegie Council on Adolescent Development

1995   *Great Transitions: Preparing Adolescents for a New Century.* Carnegie Council on Adolescent Development. New York : Carnegie Corporation of New York.

Dryfoos, J.G.

1998   *Safe Passage: Making It Through Adolescence in a Risky Society: What Parents, Schools and Communities Can Do.* New York: Oxford University Press.

Duncan, G.J., and J. Brooks-Gunn, eds.

1997   *Consequences of Growing Up Poor.* New York: Russell Sage Foundation.

Family and Child Well-Being Research Network

1999   Family and Child Well-Being Research Network. Demographic and Behavioral Sciences Branch, National Institute of Child Health and Human Development. Web site: http://famchild.wsu.edu. Contact: Demographic and Behavioral Sciences Branch, Center for Population Research, National Institute of Child Health and Human Development, 6100 Executive Blvd., Rm. 8B13, Bethesda, MD 20892. Telephone: (301) 496-1174.

Federal Interagency Forum on Child and Family Statistics

1997   *America's Children: Key National Indicators of Well-Being.* Washington, DC: Federal Interagency Forum on Child and Family Statistics.

Hauser, R.M., B.V. Brown, and W.R. Prosser, eds.

1997   *Indicators of Children's Well-Being.* New York: Russell Sage Foundation.

Moore, K.A.

1998   Criteria for indicators of child well-being. In *Indicators of Children's Well-Being.* R.M. Hauser, B.V. Brown, and W.R. Prosser, eds. New York : Russell Sage Foundation.

National Research Council

1993   *Losing Generations: Adolescents in High-Risk Settings.* Panel on High Risk Youth, National Research Council. Washington, D.C.: National Academy Press.

1996   *Youth Development and Neighborhood Influences: Challenges and Opportunities.* Committee on Youth Development. Washington, DC: National Academy Press.

Newacheck P., M. McManus, and C. Brindis

1990   Financing health care for adolescents: Problems, prospects and proposals. *Journal of Adolescent Health Care* 11(5):398-403.

Resnick, M.D., et al.

1997   Protecting adolescents from harm. Findings from the National Longitudinal Study on Adolescent Health. *Journal of the American Medical Association* 278(10):823-832.

Small, S.A.

1990   Preventive Programs That Support Families With Adolescents. Working paper of the Carnegie Council on Adolescent Development. New York : Carnegie Corporation of New York.

# Appendix
# Institute of Medicine/National Research Council Reports Relevant to Adolescence

*Adolescent Behavior and Health* (1978) summarizes the deliberations of a conference convened to examine the formation of health-relevant behavior during early adolescence.

*Adolescent Decision Making: Implications for Prevention Programs* (1999) summarizes the presentations and discussions of a workshop examining the current knowledge base regarding adolescent decision making, and the implications of this research with respect to their involvement in risk behaviors and the design of prevention interventions.

*Adolescent Development and the Biology of Puberty: Summary of a Workshop on New Research* (1999) summarizes presentations and discussions of a workshop convened to examine new research on adolescent development and the biology of puberty.

*AIDS and Behavior: An Integrated Approach* (1994) describes what investigators in the biobehavioral, psychological, and social sciences have discovered about the behavioral and mental health aspects of HIV infection and AIDS, and offers recommendations for research directions and priorities.

*Alcoholism, Alcohol Abuse and Related Problems* (1980) reviews the research field and assesses the scientific opportunities in particular areas: medical and psychological etiologies and consequences of alcohol abuse and alcoholism, the pathogenicity of alcohol, the relation of alcohol use and abuse to other major medical disorders, the development of diagnostic procedures and techniques, and the applicability of research methodologies to the development and assessment of treatment and prevention techniques.

*America's Fathers and Public Policy* (1994) summarizes the comments of participants at a workshop that addressed issues related to fathers under stress, including child support, teenage fathers, fathers of disabled children, and inner-city poor fathers, and presents selected research findings on these topics.

*America's Children: Health Insurance and Access to Care* (1998) provides an overview of key issues in the organization, delivery, and financing of health care for children, including evaluating empirical evidence about the relationship between health insurance and access to care and identifying key trends in insurance coverage and the delivery of care for uninsured children.

*Assessing the Social and Behavioral Science Base for HIV/AIDS Prevention and Intervention* (1995), a paper originally presented at an IOM workshop on the social and behavioral science base for HIV/AIDS prevention and intervention, describes a practical integrative theory on how to coordinate efforts to halt the spread of HIV/AIDS and discover knowledge gaps.

*Bereavement: Reactions, Consequences, and Care* (1984) examines the factors that affect the bereavement process and its impact on general and mental health. It covers emotional reactions and health consequences of bereavement, biological and social science perspectives on its effects, and various approaches to assisting bereaved people. The book includes a chapter on bereavement in children and adolescents.

*The Best Intentions: Unintended Pregnancy and the Well-Being of Children and Families* (1995) offers a timely exploration of family planning issues, including information on pregnancy rates and trends, the effectiveness of pregnancy prevention programs, the health and social consequences of unintended pregnancies, and the factors that shape decisions about sex, contraception, and pregnancy.

*Broadening the Base of Treatment for Alcohol Problems* (1990) reviews research and experience on alternative approaches and mechanisms for alcoholism and alcohol abuse treatment and rehabilitative services; assesses evidence on comparative costs, quality, effectiveness, and appropriateness of such services; reviews the state of financing alternatives available to the public; and makes recommendations for policies and programs of research, planning, administration, and reimbursement for treatment.

*Development During Middle Childhood: The Years from Six to Twelve* (1984) identifies significant aspects of social, emotional, cognitive, and physical development during the early elementary years, reviews the status of relevant basic research, highlights theoretical and methodological issues, and makes recommendations for future research.

*Dispelling the Myths About Addiction: Strategies to Increase Understanding and Strengthen Research* (1997) identifies and addresses barriers to public understanding of addiction, including those that present obstacles for attracting and sustaining talented investigators and other health professionals who wish to pursue careers in addiction research.

*Education and Learning to Think* (1987) addresses the question of what schools in America can do to more effectively teach what have come to be called "high-order skills." It draws conclusions about what are high-order skills, whether high-order thinking can be directly taught, and how instruction in higher-order thinking should be organized.

*Emergency Medical Services for Children* (1993) explores why emergency care for children, from infants through adolescents, must differ from that for adults and describes what seriously ill or injured children generally experience in today's systems. It makes a range of recommendations, from ensuring access through the 911 system to enhancing data resources and expanding research efforts.

*From Generation to Generation: The Health and Well-Being of Children in Immigrant Families* (1998) focuses on the fastest growing segment of the U.S. population: immigrant children and youth. It discusses the many factors—family size, fluency in English, parent employment, acculturation, delivery of health and social services, and public policies—that shape the outlook for the lives of these children, and makes recommendations for improved research and data collection designed to advance knowledge and, as a result, the visibility of these children in current policy debates.

*Growing Up Tobacco Free: Preventing Nicotine Addiction in Children and Youth* (1994) addresses the troubling issues surrounding youth and tobacco use, including explaining nicotine's effects and the process of addiction, documenting the search for an effective approach to preventing smoking, summarizing the results of recent initiatives to limit or control access and use of tobacco, and examining the controversial area of tobacco advertising.

*Health and Behavior: Frontiers of Research in Biobehavioral Sciences* (1982) briefly describes many promising directions in basic, applied, and clinical sciences that contribute to an understanding of human behavior. Coverage is broad but not exhaustive and includes a discussion of prevention efforts for adolescents related to smoking, alcohol use, marijuana use, sexual activity, diet and exercise, schooling, and delinquency.

*The Hidden Epidemic: Confronting Sexually Transmitted Diseases* (1997) examines the epidemiological dimensions of STDs in the United States and the factors that contribute to the epidemic; assesses the effectiveness of current public health strategies and programs to prevent and control STDs; and provides direction for future public health programs, policy, and research in STD prevention and control.

*Homelessness, Health, and Human Needs* (1988) is a study of the delivery of inpatient and outpatient health services to homeless people. Taking a broad view of health care and of needs for health-care-related services, including nutrition, mental health, alcohol and drug abuse problems, and dental care, it treats adolescents as a particularly vulnerable subgroup of the homeless population.

*Improving Health in the Community: A Role for Performance Monitoring* (1997) summarizes the work of a two-year study intended to examine the use of performance monitoring and develop sets of indicators that communities could use to promote the achievement of public health goals.

*Improving Schooling for Language-Minority Children* (1997) is a comprehensive review and synthesis of research on the education of limited-English-proficient and bilingual students. The book reviews a broad range of studies—from basic ones on language, literacy, and learning to others in educational settings. It proposes a research agenda that responds to issues of policy and practice while maintaining scientific integrity.

*In Her Lifetime: Female Morbidity and Mortality in Sub-Saharan Africa* (1996) provides a solid documentary base that can be used to develop an agenda to guide research and health policy formulation on female health— both for Sub-Saharan Africa and for other regions of the developing world. It covers such topics as demographics, nutritional status, obstetric morbidity and mortality, mental health problems, and sexually transmitted diseases, including HIV.

*In Her Own Right: The Institute of Medicine's Guide to Women's Health Issues* (1997) synthesizes the IOM's views on fast-moving developments in medicine in an overview of women's health across the life span, highlighting what is known about the health differences between men and woman and the mysteries that remain to be solved.

*Inner-City Poverty in the United States* (1990) documents the continuing growth of concentrated poverty in central cities and examines what is known about its causes and effects.

*Integrating Federal Statistics on Children: Report of a Workshop* (1995) summarizes a meeting held to examine the adequacy of federal statistics on children and families against a framework of key developmental transition points in the lives of children and adolescents.

*Losing Generations: Adolescents in High-Risk Settings* (1993) explores the settings in which American youths are expected to mature into responsible adulthood, including families, schools, and communities, and illuminates the challenging policy issues that decision makers face in this realm.

*Neither Angels Nor Thieves: Studies in Deinstitutionalization of Status Offenders* (1982) examines what happened to youth who committed status offenses (e.g., truants, runaways, incorrigibles) in the aftermath of the 1974 Juvenile Justice and Delinquency Prevention Act. The legislation mandated the removal of these youth from secure confinement, prohibited their subsequent incarceration, and called for the development of alternative types of community-based programs and services. The report includes analyses of state and federal program based on field work in 7 states and 14 local areas.

*The New Americans: Economic, Demographic, and Fiscal Effects of Immigration* (1997) sheds light on one of the most controversial issues of the decade, identifying the economic gains and losses from immigration for the country, states, and localities, and providing a foundation for public discussion and policy making.

*New Findings on Poverty and Child Health and Nutrition* (1998) summarizes a workshop at which researchers presented recent findings in the areas of poverty, child health, and nutrition, highlighting key findings relevant to the contemporary debate about welfare and health care policy for the poor, and examining priorities for future research that will yield insights into the effects of welfare reform. The report also features a discussion of state and local officials' data and research needs, and examples of new child health interventions and projects monitoring the effects of welfare reform.

*New Findings on Welfare and Children's Development: Summary of a Research Briefing* (1994) presents research on how children and youth are affected by growing up in families that receive welfare benefits.

*Pathways of Addiction: Opportunities in Drug Abuse Research* (1996) provides a national research agenda designed to yield the greatest benefit from limited resources. The book covers the epidemiology and etiology of drug abuse and discusses several of its most troubling health and social consequences, including HIV, violence, and harm to children, as well as the efficacy of preventive interventions and treatments.

*Paying Attention to Children in a Changing Health Care System* (1996) summarizes five workshops convened between 1991 and 1994 to explore various aspects of maternal and child health care in an era of health system change.

*Preventing Drug Abuse: What Do We Know?* (1993) provides a comprehensive overview of what is known about drug abuse prevention and its effectiveness, including results of a range of antidrug efforts; a profile of the drug problem, including a look at drug use by different population groups; an exploration of three schools of prevention theory; a view of the role and effectiveness of mass media in preventing drug use; and an examination of promising prevention techniques.

*Protecting Youth at Work: Health, Safety, and Development of Working Children and Adolescents in the United States* (1999) assesses what is known about work done in the United States by children and adolescents and the effects of that work on their physical and emotional health and social functioning. It presents a wide range of data and analysis on the scope of youth employment, factors that put children and adolescents at risk in the workplace, and the positive and negative effects of employment, including data on educational attainment and lifestyle choices.

*Reducing Risks for Mental Disorders: Frontiers for Preventive Intervention Research* (1994) reviews advances in understanding of how to reduce risk factors for mental disorders in the context of current research, and provides a targeted definition of prevention and a conceptual framework that emphasizes risk reduction. The report includes a focused research agenda with recommendations on how to develop effective intervention programs, create a cadre of prevention researchers, and improve coordination among government agencies and private foundations.

*Reproductive Health in Developing Countries: Expanding Dimensions, Building Solutions* (1997) assesses the magnitude and severity of reproductive health problems in developing countries, examines the likely costs and effectiveness of interventions to improve reproductive health, and recommends priorities for programs, research, and data collection.

*Research on Children and Adolescents with Mental, Behavioral, and Developmental Disorders* (1989) examines the status of research on emotional, behavioral, and developmental mental disorders in children and adolescents. It documents the progress being made in understanding, preventing, and treating such disorders, highlights some of the many promising opportunities for future research, and delineates critical resource requirements for advancing the field.

*Research on Mental Illness and Addictive Disorders: Progress and Prospects* (1984) summarizes progress in understanding, preventing, and treating mental and addictive disorders (including depression and mania, schizophrenia, anxiety and phobias, drug abuse, alcoholism, personality disorders, severe mental disorders of childhood and old age, and the problems of chronic mental illness), and highlights promising directions for further advances.

*Risking the Future: Adolescent Sexuality, Pregnancy, and Childbearing* (1987) examines data on trends in teenage sexuality and fertility behavior, reviews and synthesizes research on the antecedents and consequences of early pregnancy and childbearing, and reviews alternative preventive and ameliorative policies and programs. It includes discussion of priorities for data collection and research.

*Schools and Health: Our Nation's Investment* (1997), the report of an IOM committee charged with studying K-12 comprehensive school health programs, provides a framework for determining desirable and feasible health outcomes of such programs, examines the relationship between health and education outcomes, considers factors necessary to optimize these outcomes, appraises data on effectiveness, and recommends ways to implement effective school-based health programs.

*Sleeping Pills, Insomnia, and Medical Practice* (1979) reviews both clinical issues and public health problems associated with the prescribing of sleeping pills (hypnotics) containing secobarbital, pentobarbital, and amobarbital. The report includes a discussion of suicide and accidental overdose, traffic safety, and nonmedical use related to these drugs.

*Social Dynamics of Adolescent Fertility in Sub-Saharan Africa* (1993) is one of a series of reports on the population dynamics of Sub-Saharan Africa. This report describes the changing social context within which adolescents are having children in Sub-Saharan Africa, and the effects of these changing circumstances on the benefits and risks of early childbearing.

*Social Marketing to Adolescent and Minority Populations: Workshop Summary* (1995) summarizes ideas about the use and effectiveness of social marketing in communicating health promotion and disease prevention information to adolescent and minority populations, summarizes the limited evaluative information available on social marketing to these populations, and suggests questions for future research.

*Systems of Accountability: Implementing Children's Health Insurance Programs*

(1998) addresses practical concerns about the implementation and evaluation of the State Children's Health Insurance Program, and presents recommendations about accountability for measuring the program's impact.

*Taking Action to Reduce Tobacco Use* (1998) addresses tobacco control in terms of price increases, federal regulation, state and local tobacco control programs, performance monitoring, cessation programs, research, and international health impacts.

*Transitions in Work and Learning: Implications for Assessment* (1997) provides a conceptual framework and empirical base necessary for inquiry into the pressing issues surrounding transitions into and between learning and work environments.

*Treating Drug Problems: A Study of the Evolution, Effectiveness, and Financing of Public and Private Drug Treatment Systems* (1990) discusses the history of ideas governing drug policy, the nature and extent of the need for treatment, the goals and effectiveness of treatment, the need for research on treatment methods and services, the costs and organization of the two-tiered national treatment system, the scope and organizing principles of public and private coverage, and provides recommendations tailored to each kind of coverage.

*2020 Vision: Health in the 21st Century* (1996), published on the 25th anniversary of the Institute of Medicine, explores the challenges of the coming 25 years with an eye to the forces that will affect Americans' lives, health, and health care system.

*Understanding Child Abuse and Neglect* (1993) includes a comprehensive overview of definitions and the scope of child maltreatment, an examination of research on the causes, consequences, treatment, and prevention of child abuse and neglect, and a discussion of the human and other resources needed to move research in this area forward.

*Understanding Risk: Informing Decisions in a Democratic Society* (1996) addresses a central dilemma of coping with risk in a democracy: detailed scientific and technical information is essential for making decisions, but the people who make and live with those decisions are not scientists. It argues that making risks understandable to the public involves much more than just translating scientific information.

*Understanding Violence against Women* (1996) is a comprehensive overview of current knowledge in the area of violence against women and identifies four areas with the greatest potential for increasing understanding of domestic violence and rape: (1) what interventions are designed to do; (2) factors that put people at risk of violence and that precipitate violence; (3) the scope of domestic violence and sexual assault in America and its consequences to individuals, families, and society; and (4) how to structure the study of violence to yield more useful knowledge.

*Urban Change and Poverty* (1988) describes the uncertainties facing cities and their economies and populations, identifies the urban policy issues facing state, local, and federal policy makers, and assesses possible policy responses at each level of the intergovernmental system. It includes background papers on a set of specific issues.

*Violence and the American Family* (1994) summarizes discussions from a workshop held to identify key issues to be addressed in responding to the problem of family violence, determine the state of research in the field, and consider the nexus between research and policy initiatives.

*Violence in Families: Assessing Prevention and Treatment Programs* (1998) provides a comprehensive review of the successes and failures of family violence interventions; offers recommendations to guide services, programs, policy, and research; and outlines new strategies for researcher-practitioner collaboration that can improve the design and evaluation of prevention and treatment services; the report also features an analysis of 114 evaluation studies on the outcomes of different kinds of programs and services.

*Violence in Urban America: Mobilizing a Response* (1994) summarizes a conference convened to communicate the information contained in several reports on violence and, in combination with experience from practice, to identify new approaches to and interventions against various manifestations of violence.

*Volunteers in Public Schools* (1990) is an overview of volunteer activity in U.S. public schools—how volunteers are being used, what factors make programs successful, what further research will enhance the ability to create effective programs, and what directions national policy should take. It includes reports of site visits to 13 "exemplary" programs.

*Youth Development and Neighborhood Influences: Challenges and Opportunities* (1996) reports on a workshop that focused on what is known about environmental influences that interact with youth characteristics, family factors, and peer influences to foster or inhibit successful outcomes for adolescents; the report describes processes for community and family interactions during periods of adolescent development, reviews the literature on social settings and youth development, and touches on selected community youth service programs.

# Other Reports from the Board on Children, Youth, and Families

*Adolescent Development and the Biology of Puberty: Summary of a Workshop on New Research* (1999)

*Adolescent Decision Making: Implications for Prevention Programs: Summary of a Workshop* (1999)

*Protecting Youth at Work: Health, Safety, and Development of Working Children and Adolescents in the United States* (1998)

*America's Children: Health Insurance and Access to Care* (with the IOM Division of Health Care Services) (1998)

*Systems of Accountability: Implementing Children's Health Insurance Programs* (with the IOM Division of Health Care Services) (1998)

*Longitudinal Surveys of Children: Report of a Workshop* (with the NRC Committee on National Statistics) (1998)

*From Generation to Generation: The Health and Well-Being of Children in Immigrant Families* (1998)

*New Findings on Poverty and Child Health and Nutrition: Summary of a Research Briefing* (1998)

*Violence in Families: Assessing Treatment and Prevention Programs,* 1998

*Welfare, the Family, and Reproductive Behavior: Report of a Meeting* (with the NRC Committee on Population) (1998)

*Educating Language-Minority Children* (1998)

*Improving Schooling for Language-Minority Children: A Research Agenda* (1997)

*New Findings on Welfare and Children's Development: Summary of a Research Briefing* (1997)

*Youth Development and Neighborhood Influences: Challenges and Opportunities: Summary of a Workshop* (1996)

*Paying Attention to Children in a Changing Health Care System: Summaries of Workshops* (1996)

*Integrating Federal Statistics on Children* (with the NRC Committee on National Statistics) (1995)